It's easy to get lost in the cancer world

Let NCCN Guidelines for Patients® be your guide

- Step-by-step guides to the cancer care options likely to have the best results
- Based on treatment guidelines used by health care providers worldwide
- Designed to help you discuss cancer treatment with your doctors

National Comprehensive Cancer Network®

NCCN Guidelines for Patients® are developed by the National Comprehensive Cancer Network® (NCCN®)

NCCN

- An alliance of leading cancer centers across the United States devoted to patient care, research, and education

Cancer centers that are part of NCCN: NCCN.org/cancercenters

NCCN Clinical Practice Guidelines in Oncology (NCCN Guidelines®)

- Developed by doctors from NCCN cancer centers using the latest research and years of experience
- For providers of cancer care all over the world
- Expert recommendations for cancer screening, diagnosis, and treatment

Free online at NCCN.org/guidelines

NCCN Guidelines for Patients

- Present information from the NCCN Guidelines in an easy-to-learn format
- For people with cancer and those who support them
- Explain the cancer care options likely to have the best results

Free online at NCCN.org/patientguidelines

NATIONAL COMPREHENSIVE CANCER NETWORK FOUNDATION
Guiding Treatment. Changing Lives.

and supported by funding from NCCN Foundation®

These NCCN Guidelines for Patients are based on the NCCN Guidelines® for Bone Cancer (Version 1.2021, November 20, 2020).

NCCN Foundation seeks to support the millions of patients and their families affected by a cancer diagnosis by funding and distributing NCCN Guidelines for Patients. NCCN Foundation is also committed to advancing cancer treatment by funding the nation's promising doctors at the center of innovation in cancer research. For more details and the full library of patient and caregiver resources, visit NCCN.org/patients.

National Comprehensive Cancer Network (NCCN) / NCCN Foundation
3025 Chemical Road, Suite 100
Plymouth Meeting, PA 19462
215.690.0300

Endorsed by

Northwest Sarcoma Foundation

Our mission: To provide hope, education, and support to sarcoma patients and their families in the Pacific Northwest while investing in research to improve cure rates for sarcomas. nwsarcoma.org

SARC

Sarcoma advocacy is integral to the mission of SARC and to our community. Together, we are working to help build awareness of sarcoma and the resources that are available to help patients and their families. sarctrials org.

The Alan B. Slifka Foundation

Founded in 1965, the Alan B. Slifka Foundation is a private family foundation dedicated to the pursuit of inclusion, diversity, peace and healing. The Foundation seeks to combat cancer, especially childhood cancer, through the support of innovative biomedical research. Among the Foundation's top priorities is funding research into less toxic, more effective and potentially curative therapies for a variety of cancers, but especially for connective tissue cancers, known as sarcomas, that disproportionately impact children and young adults. The Alan B. Slifka Foundation is particularly interested in supporting bench-to-bedside research that results in targeted therapies, and also research that enhances our understanding of the metastatic process.slifkafoundation.org

The Paula Takacs Foundation

The mission of the Paula Takacs Foundation for Sarcoma Research is to raise funds that will directly benefit the fight to eradicate sarcomas. By supporting local, innovative research with a relentless commitment to excellence, we open a pathway for scientists and other research professionals to develop and offer cutting-edge treatment options to more sarcoma sufferers. Thus, helping to expand global hope for cures.

paulatakacsfoundation.org

The QuadW Foundation

The QuadW Foundation provides financial support to people and organizations pursuing innovative ideas and opportunities in the areas of higher education, sarcoma research, personally transforming mission experiences and general philanthropy. Our accomplishments will reflect the light-hearted but whole-hearted spirit that Willie embodied. quadw.org

With generous support from

Warren Chow, MD

To make a gift or learn more, please visit NCCNFoundation.org/donate
or e-mail PatientGuidelines@nccn.org.

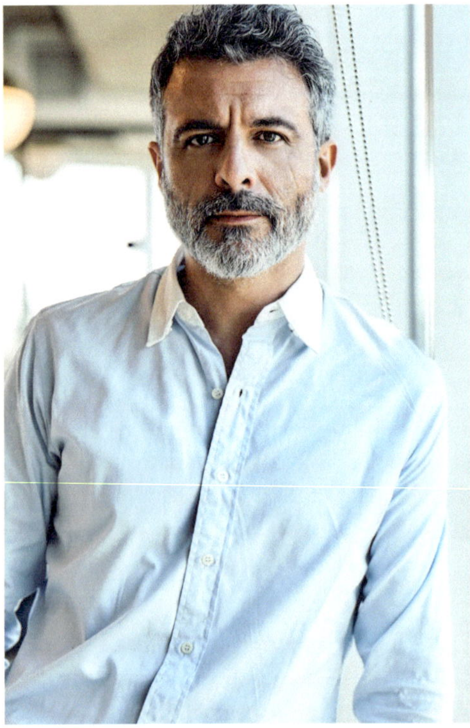
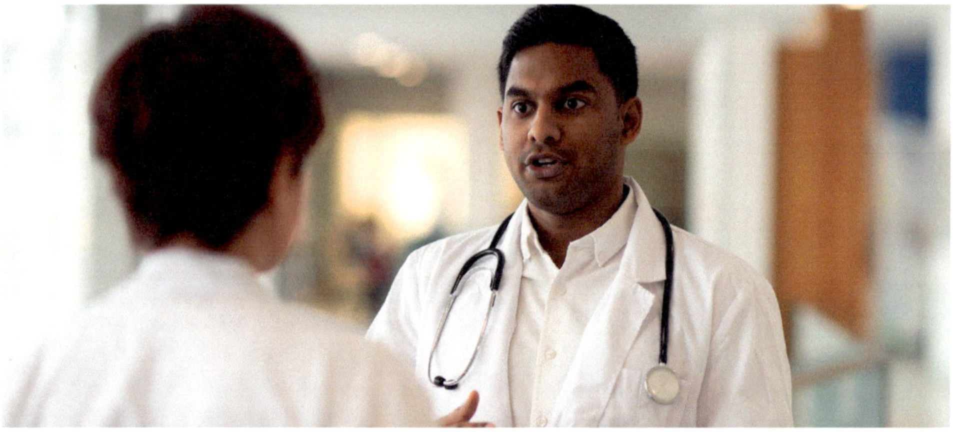
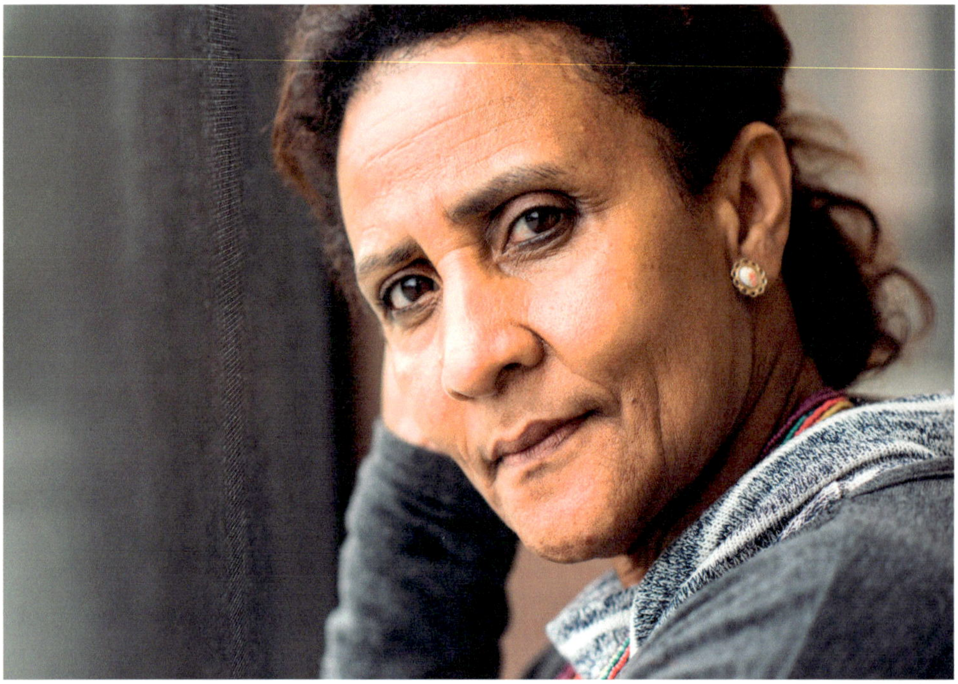
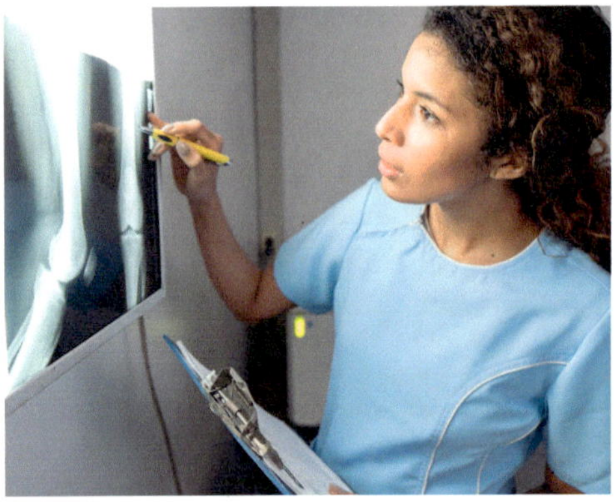
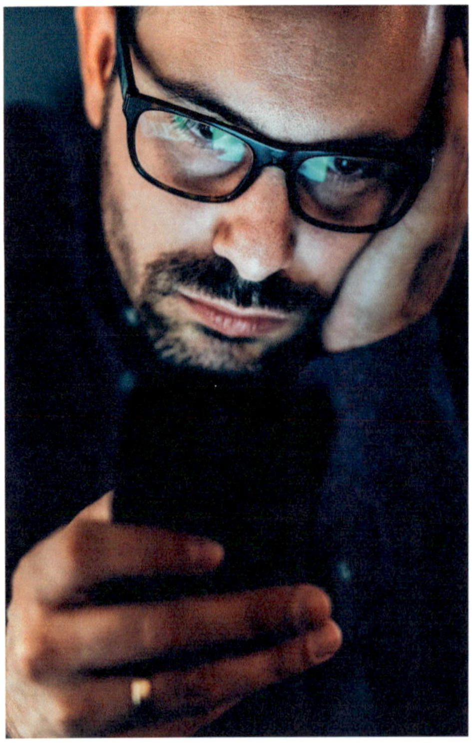
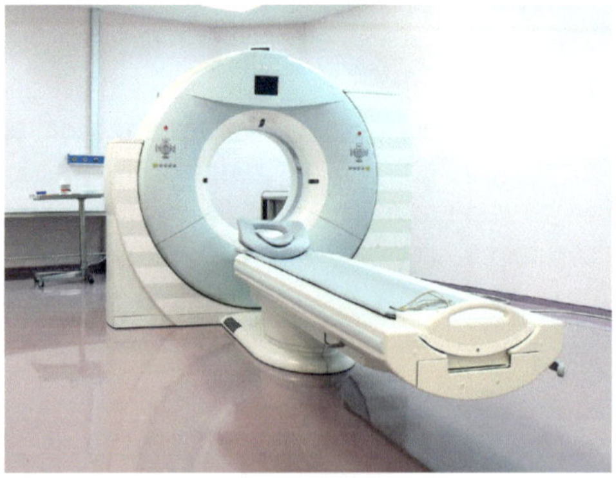
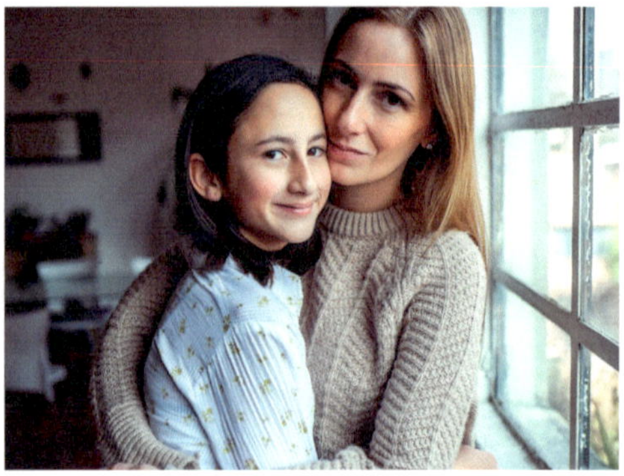
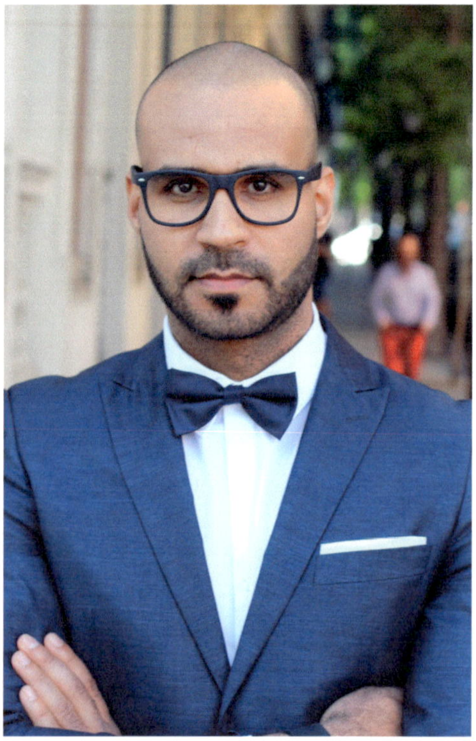

Contents

1
The bone

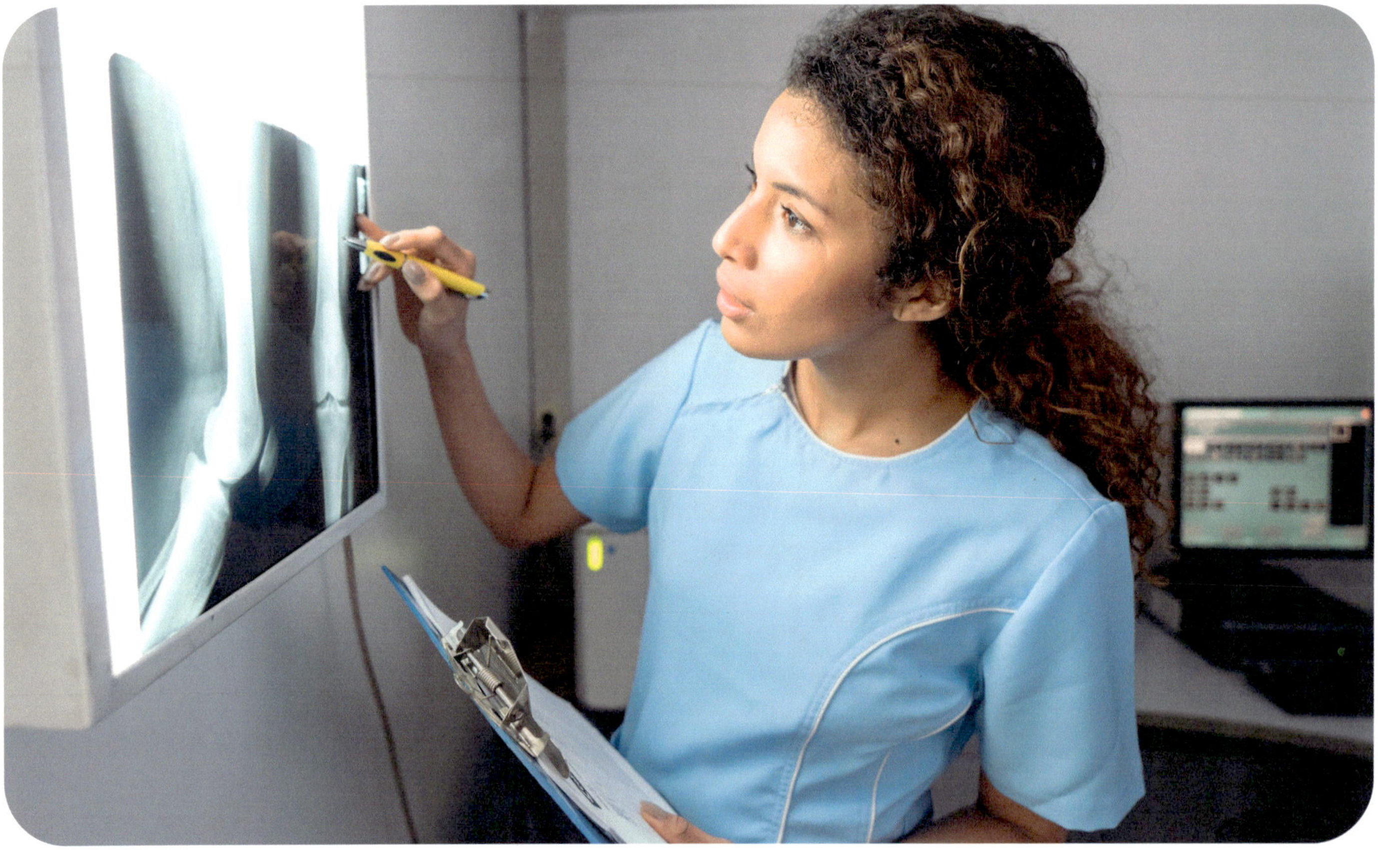

Bone cancer includes a group of cancers that start in the bone or cartilage. This is called primary bone cancer and differs from other cancers that can spread or metastasize to the bone. This chapter presents an overview of bone cancer.

The bone

Bone is a living tissue made up of collagen. Collagen is the most abundant protein in the body. Bone tissue also contains blood vessels, nerves, proteins, vitamins, and minerals.

Our body has about 206 bones. Bones provide structure and support, protect our organs, create blood cells, store chemicals the body needs, and produce hormones. Bone is light, yet strong and can regrow.

Bone is made up of the following:

- Compact tissue - the hard, outer layer that is covered by a membrane of connective tissue called the periosteum
- Cancellous tissue - the spongy, inner layer that contains red marrow
- Bone marrow - found in the center of most bones and has many blood vessels. There are 2 types of bone marrow: red and yellow. Red marrow contains blood stem cells that can become red blood cells, white blood cells, or platelets. Yellow marrow is made mostly of fat.

The skeletal system

The human skeletal system consists of bones, cartilage, ligaments, and tendons. It includes all of the bones and joints in the body.

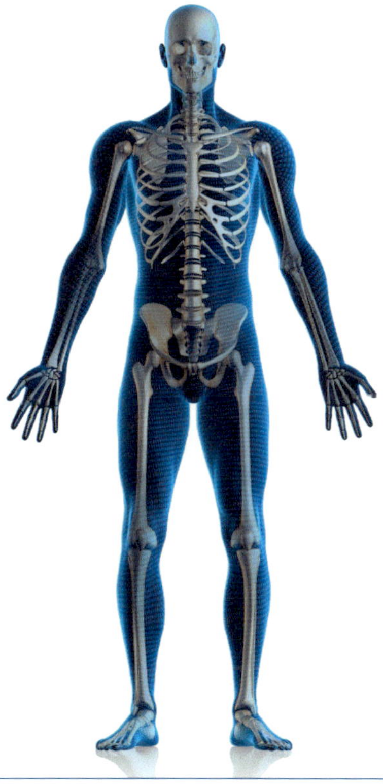

How bone is formed

New bone formation or ossification starts in the womb and ends during adolescence, between the ages of 10 and 19 years of age.

There are 2 forms of ossification:

- Compact bone (endochondral), which makes up most of the skeleton
- Cancellous bone (intermembranous), which includes parts of the skull, the shoulder blades, and the ends of the long bones. Long bones are longer than they are wide.

Once ossification is complete, bone is replaced during a remodeling process. Remodeling maintains normal calcium levels in the body. When calcium is needed, cells called osteoclasts break down bone. This releases calcium into the bloodstream. At the same time, bone-forming cells called osteoblasts create bone. Some types of bone cancer can interrupt this process.

There are 3 parts to bone:

- Epiphysis - the end of the bone
- Metaphysis - located between the physis (growth plate) and diaphysis
- Diaphysis - the middle region of the bone

The type of bone cancer is often based on where it is found in the bone.

Anatomy of the bone

There are 3 parts to the bone. The epiphysis is the end of the bone. The metaphysis is located between the physis (growth plate) and the diaphysis. The diaphysis is the middle region of the bone.

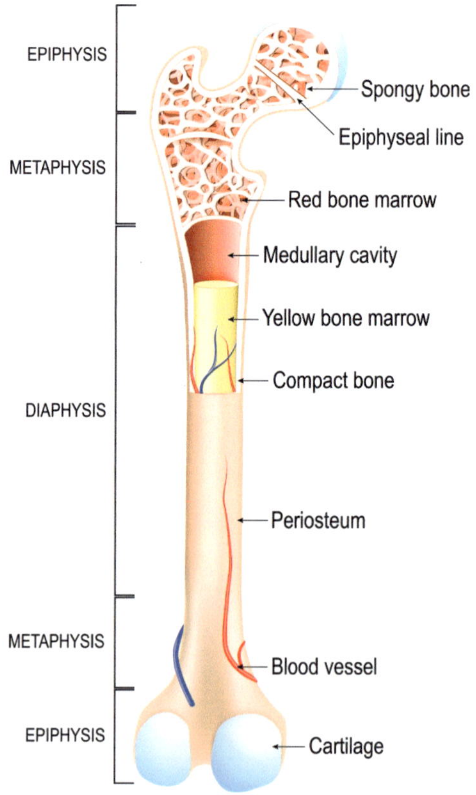

Types of bone tumors

A bone tumor is an abnormal growth of cells within a bone. A bone tumor may be cancerous (malignant) or noncancerous (benign). The cause of bone tumors is unknown. They often occur in areas of the bone that grow rapidly.

This book will discuss the following:

- Chondrosarcoma – starts in the cells that form cartilage. Cartilage is a tough, flexible tissue that lines joints and gives structure to the nose, ears, larynx, and other parts of the body.
- Chordoma - starts in notochordal cells that form the spine and vertebrae. Chordomas are usually found in the lower spinal column or at the base of the skull.
- Ewing sarcoma – starts in the marrow and commonly occurs in the diaphysis.
- Giant cell tumor of the bone (GCTB) – is an overgrowth of cells found in the epiphysis.
- Osteosarcoma – starts in cells that form bone in the metaphysis and some growth plates.

Since bone cancer is very rare, many doctors are not experts in diagnosing or treating these tumors. Therefore, it is important to find a treatment center or hospital that has both experts and experience in your type of bone cancer.

Bone cancer

Cancers that start in the bone are called primary bone tumors. Bone cancers that start in another part of the body (such as the breast, lungs, or colon) are called secondary or metastatic bone tumors. They behave very differently from primary bone tumors.

Sarcomas

Most bone cancers are sarcomas. Sarcomas are a rare group of cancers.

There are 2 main types of sarcomas:

- Soft tissue
- Bone

Soft tissue includes fat, muscles, nerves, tendons, blood and lymph vessels, and other supportive tissues of the body. Soft tissue sarcomas are more common than bone sarcomas. Bone sarcomas, such as osteosarcomas, start in the cells that form bone. Osteosarcoma, Ewing sarcoma, and chondrosarcoma are the most common types of bone cancer.

The *NCCN Guidelines for Patients: Soft Tissue Sarcoma* can be found at NCCN.org/patientguidelines.

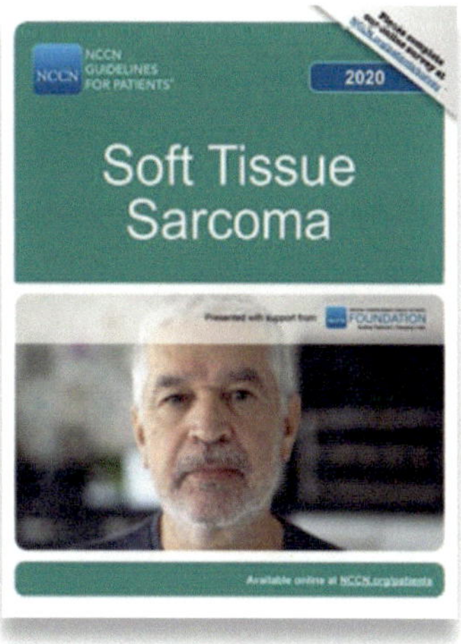

How bone cancer spreads

Unlike normal cells, cancer cells can grow or spread to form tumors in other parts of the body. This is called a metastasis.

Cancer can spread through blood or the lymphatic system. The lymphatic system contains a clear fluid called lymph. Lymph gives cells water and food and contains white blood cells that fight germs. Lymph nodes filter lymph and remove the germs. Lymph travels throughout the body in vessels like blood does. Lymph vessels and nodes are found everywhere in the body. Although cancer can spread through your blood, you cannot spread your cancer to other people if they are exposed to your blood.

Bone cancer can spread to the lung or other bones. Bone cancer that has metastasized to the lung is still called bone cancer.

Types of sarcoma

There are many types of sarcoma. This image shows only some types of sarcoma.

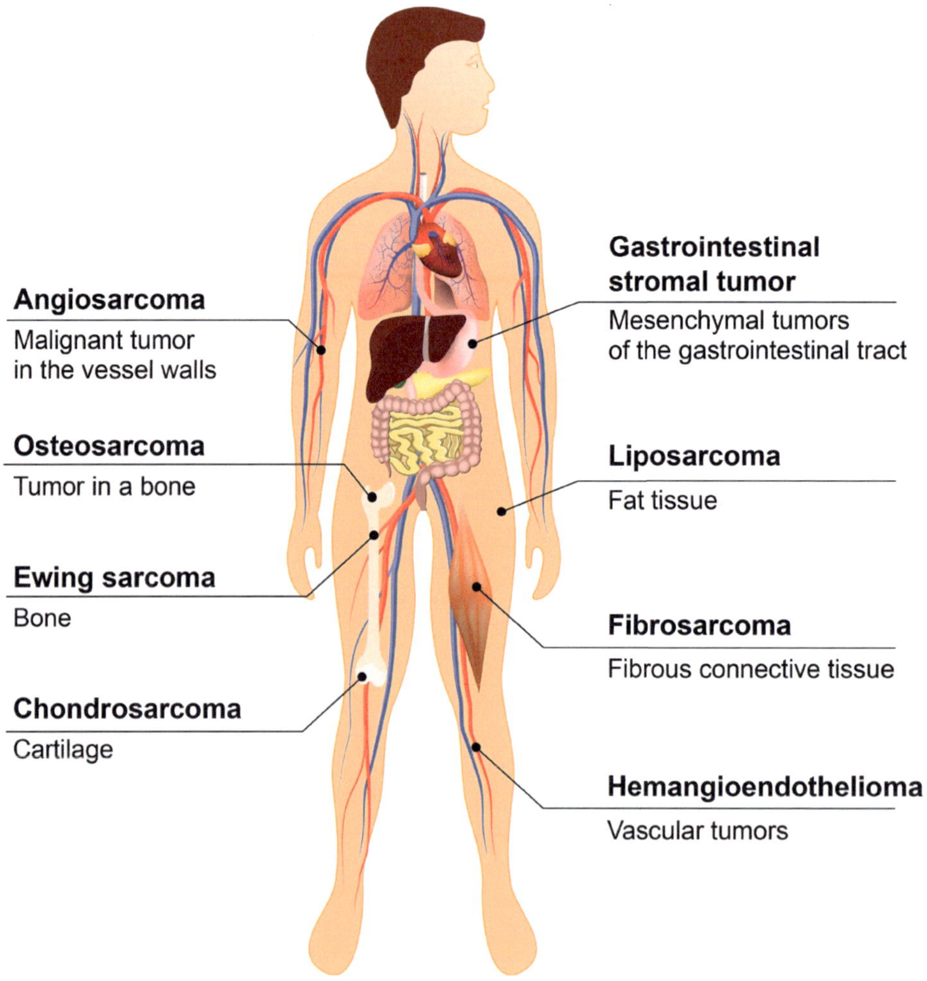

Review

- Bone cancer is a group of cancers that start in the bone or cartilage. This is called primary bone cancer. Bone cancers that start in another part of the body (such as the breast, lungs, or colon) are called secondary or metastatic bone tumors.
- Bone tumors may be cancerous (malignant) or noncancerous (benign). The cause of bone tumors is unknown.
- Bone sarcomas, such as osteosarcomas, start in the cells that form bone. Most bone cancers are sarcomas.
- Osteosarcoma, Ewing sarcoma, and chondrosarcoma are the most common types of bone cancer.
- Bone cancer can metastasize to the lungs and other bones.
- It is important to find a treatment center or hospital that has both experts and experience in your type of bone cancer.

Those with bone cancer should be treated by a team of doctors from different fields of medicine who have knowledge and experience with your type of cancer.

2

Testing for bone cancer

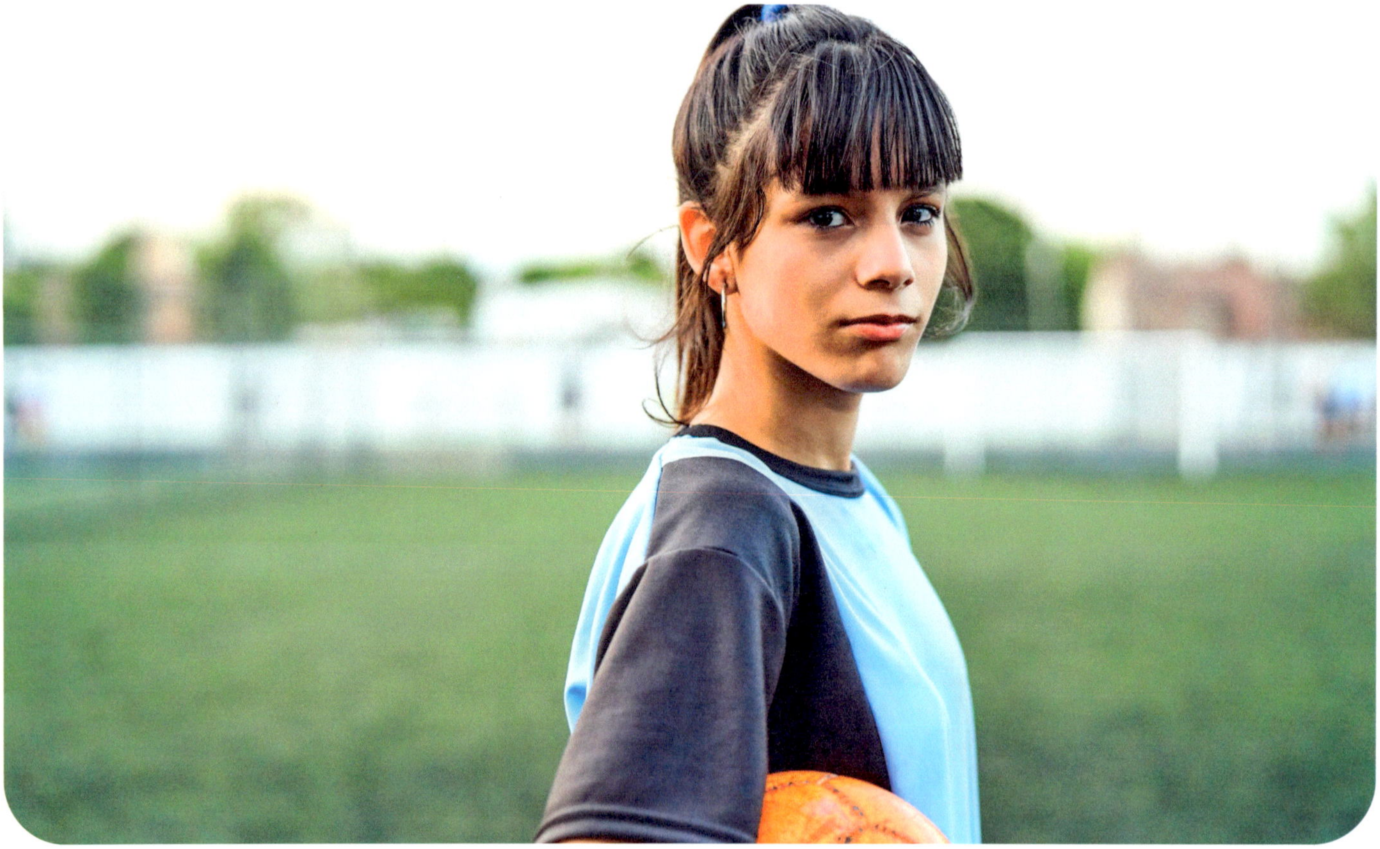

Treatment planning starts with testing. Accurate testing is needed to diagnose and treat bone cancer. A biopsy is recommended before starting treatment. This chapter presents an overview of the tests you might receive and what to expect.

Test results

Results from blood and tissue tests, imaging studies, and biopsy will determine your treatment plan. It is important you understand what these tests mean. Ask questions and keep copies of your test results. Online patient portals are a great way to access your test results.

Whether you are going for a second opinion, test, or office visit, keep these things in mind:

- Bring someone with you to doctor visits, if possible.
- Write down questions and take notes during appointments. Don't be afraid to ask your care team questions. Get to know your care team and let them get to know you.
- Get copies of blood tests, imaging results, and reports about the specific type of cancer you have. It will be helpful when getting a second opinion.
- Organize your papers. Create files for insurance forms, medical records, and test results. You can do the same on your computer.
- Keep a list of contact information for everyone on your care team. Add it to your binder or notebook. Hang the list on your fridge or keep it by the phone.

General health tests

Medical history

A medical history is a record of all health issues and treatments you have had in your life. Be prepared to list any illness or injury and when it happened. Bring a list of old and new medicines and any over-the-counter medicines, herbals, or supplements you take. Tell your doctor about any symptoms you have. A medical history will help determine which treatment is best for you.

Family history

Some cancers and other diseases can run in families. Your doctor will ask about the health history of family members who are blood relatives. This information is called a family history. Ask family members about their health issues like heart disease, cancer, and diabetes, and at what age they were diagnosed.

Physical exam

During a physical exam a health care provider may:

- Check your temperature, blood pressure, pulse, and breathing rate
- Weigh you
- Listen to your lungs and heart
- Look in your eyes, ears, nose, and throat
- Feel and apply pressure to parts of your body to see if organs are of normal size, are soft or hard, or cause pain when touched. Tell your doctor if you feel pain.
- Feel for enlarged lymph nodes in your neck, underarm, and groin. Tell the doctor if you have felt any lumps or have any pain.
- Examine your skeletal system
- Assess your ability to manage tasks and activities that are used in daily life called a functional assessment

For possible tests, see Guide 1.

Guide 1 Testing for bone cancer: Those 40 years of age and over
Medical history and physical exam
Bone scan or PET/CT
Chest x-ray
Blood tests include serum protein electrophoresis (SPEP), complete blood count (CBC), comprehensive metabolic panel (CMP) with calcium to assess for hypercalcemia
Chest/abdominal/pelvic CT with contrast
Prostate-specific antigen (PSA)
Mammogram
Biopsy, as needed

* Those under 40 years of age will be referred to an orthopedic oncologist

Pregnancy and fertility

Bone cancer survivors are at risk for fertility issues. Fertility is the ability to have children. If you think you want children in the future, ask your doctor how cancer and cancer treatment will change your fertility and sexual health. In order to preserve your fertility, you may need to take action before starting cancer treatment.

Those who want to have children in the future should be referred to a fertility specialist before starting treatment to discuss the options. More information can be found in the *NCCN Guidelines for Patients®: Adolescents and Young Adults with Cancer*, available at NCCN.org/patientguidelines.

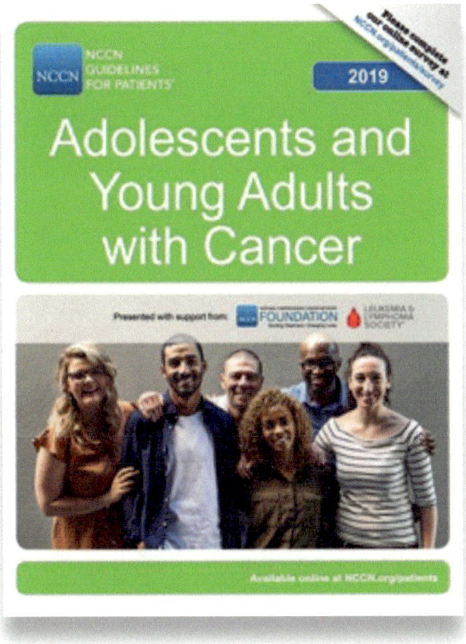

Those with ovaries

Those who can have children will have a pregnancy test before starting treatment. Cancer treatment can hurt the baby if you are or become pregnant during treatment. Therefore, birth control to prevent pregnancy during and after treatment is recommended. Hormonal birth control may not be recommended, so ask your doctor about options.

Those with testicles

Cancer and cancer treatment can damage sperm. Therefore, use contraception (birth control) to prevent pregnancy during and after cancer treatment. If you think you want children in the future, talk to your doctor now. Sperm banking is an option.

Infertility

Infertility is the complete loss of the ability to have children. The actual risk of infertility is related to your age at time of diagnosis, treatment type(s), treatment dose, and treatment length. Chemotherapy with alkylating agents has a higher risk of infertility. Sometimes, there isn't time for fertility preservation before you start treatment. Talk to your doctor about your concerns.

Pregnancy test

Those who can become pregnant will be given a pregnancy test before treatment begins.

Blood tests

Blood tests check for signs of disease and how well organs are working. They require a sample of your blood, which is removed through a needle placed into your vein. Blood tests should be done before starting treatment.

Complete blood count

A complete blood count (CBC) measures the levels of red blood cells, white blood cells, and platelets in your blood. Your doctor will want to know if you have enough red blood cells to carry oxygen throughout your body, white blood cells to fight infection, and platelets to control bleeding.

Chemistry profile

The liver, bone, and other organs release chemicals in your blood. A chemistry profile measures these levels. Abnormal results may be a sign that organs such as your liver or kidneys aren't working well. This test may be repeated during and after treatment.

A chemistry profile will look for higher than normal calcium levels in your blood called hypercalcemia. Calcium is the most common mineral in the body. It is needed for healthy teeth, bones, and other body tissues. Bone damage from cancer can cause your bones to release calcium into the bloodstream.

ALP

Alkaline phosphatase (ALP) is an enzyme found in the blood. High levels of ALP levels can be a sign of bone tumors, liver disorders, or pregnancy.

Lactic acid

Lactate dehydrogenase (LDH) or lactic acid dehydrogenase is an enzyme found in most cells. Dying cells release LDH into blood. Fast-growing cells, such as tumor cells, also release LDH.

PSA

Prostate-specific antigen (PSA) is a protein made by the fluid-making cells that line the small glands inside the prostate. Normal prostate cells, as well as prostate cancer cells, make PSA. PSA levels might be checked to detect prostate cancer, which can spread to bones.

SPEP

Serum protein electrophoresis (SPEP) examines specific proteins in the blood called globulins, which may be increased in certain conditions such as multiple myeloma.

Imaging tests

Imaging tests take pictures (images) of the inside of your body. These tests are used to look for cancer in organs and areas outside of the blood. A radiologist, an expert in test images, will write a report and send this report to your doctor. Your doctor will discuss the results with you.

X-ray

An x-ray is a type of radiation. In small doses, it is used to make pictures of the inside of the body. It might be referred to as a radiograph.

Bone scan

A bone scan uses a radiotracer to make pictures of the inside of bones. A radiotracer is a substance that releases small amounts of radiation. Before the pictures are taken, the tracer will be injected into your vein. It can take a few hours for the tracer to enter your bones.

A special camera will take pictures of the tracer in your bones. Areas of bone damage use more radiotracer than healthy bone and show up as bright spots on the pictures.

CT scan

A computed tomography (CT or CAT) scan uses x-rays and computer technology to take pictures of the inside of the body. It takes many x-rays of the same body part from different angles. All the images are combined to make one detailed picture. In most cases, contrast will be used. Contrast materials are not dyes, but substances that help certain areas in the body stand out. It is used to make the pictures clearer. The contrast is not permanent and will leave the body in your urine.

Tell your doctors if you have had bad reactions to contrast in the past. This is important. You might be given medicines, such as Benadryl® and prednisone, for an allergy to contrast. Contrast might not be used if you have a serious allergy or if your kidneys aren't working well.

MRI scan

A magnetic resonance imaging (MRI) scan uses radio waves and powerful magnets to take pictures of the inside of the body. It does not use x-rays. Contrast might be used.

PET scan

A positron emission tomography (PET) scan uses a radioactive drug called a tracer. A tracer is a substance injected into a vein to see where it is in the body and if it is using sugar to grow. Cancer cells show up as bright spots on PET scans. Not all bright spots are cancer. It is normal for the brain, heart, kidneys, and bladder to be bright on PET.

Sometimes, PET is combined with CT. This combined test is called a PET/CT scan.

Head-to-toe PET/CT

Your doctor might request a head-to-toe or whole body PET/CT. Whole-body imaging means from the top of the head through the bottom of the feet. A typical scan is from the eyes to thighs.

Mammogram

A mammogram is a picture of the insides of your breast. The pictures are made using x-rays. A computer combines the x-rays to make detailed pictures. Diagnostic mammograms are made with more x-rays than screening mammograms. A bilateral mammogram includes pictures of both breasts. It is used to identify any tumors, and if so, the number and size of the tumor(s). A mammogram might be needed to confirm that the cancer found in your bones is not from breast cancer.

Biopsy

A biopsy is the removal of a sample of tissue or group of cells for testing. A diagnosis of bone cancer is confirmed using a core needle or surgical biopsy. The placement of the biopsy is critical. Therefore, it is recommended that the biopsy be performed at an experienced center where you will receive treatment.

- Core needle biopsy removes tissue samples with a hollow needle about the same size as a needle used for an IV (intravenous) line.
- Surgical biopsy removes a piece of the tumor to be tested.

CT machine

A CT machine is large and has a tunnel in the middle. During the test, you will lie on a table that moves slowly through the tunnel.

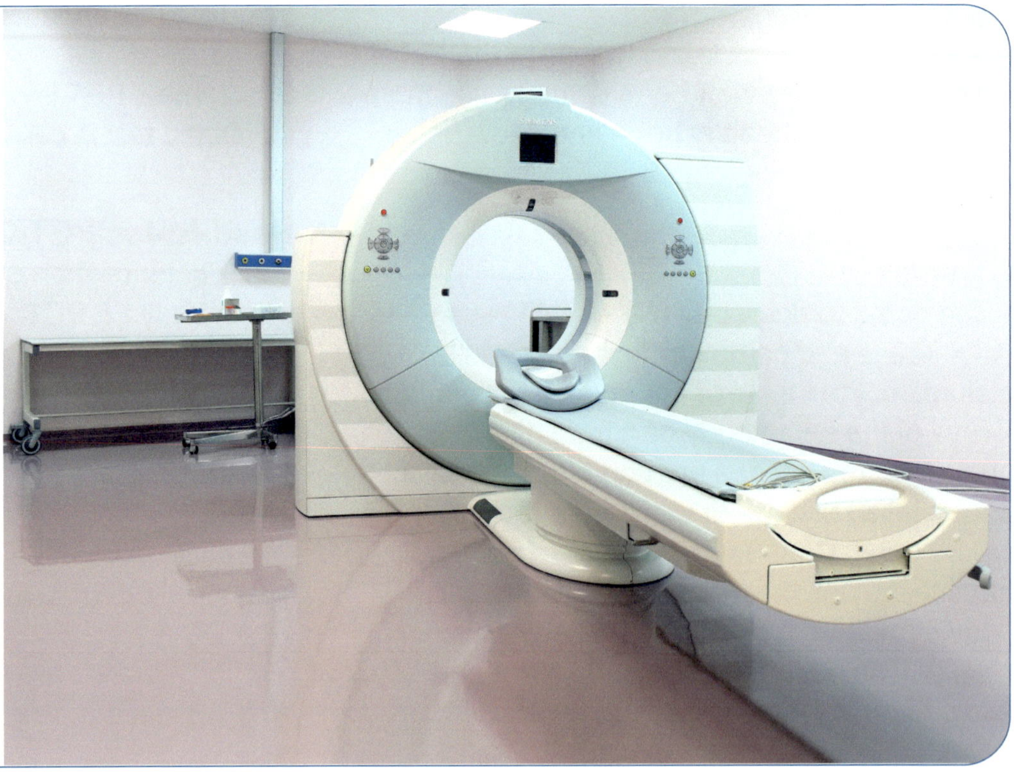

Genetic tests

Inside our cells are deoxyribonucleic acid (DNA) molecules. These molecules are tightly packaged into what is called a chromosome. Chromosomes contain most of the genetic information in a cell. Normal human cells contain 23 pairs of chromosomes for a total of 46 chromosomes. Each chromosome contains thousands of genes. Genes tell cells what to do and what to become.

There are different types of genetic tests; some are done on molecules or proteins, some on genes, and some on chromosomes. Genetic testing might include cytogenetics or molecular testing. Cytogenetics is the study of chromosomes. Cytogenetics involves testing samples of blood, tissue, and bone marrow to look for broken, missing, re-arranged, or extra chromosomes. Molecular or biomarker testing looks for specific proteins or molecules.

Ewing sarcoma

A cell must make a copy of its chromosomes before dividing into two cells. Sometimes, there are mistakes in the copies. One type of mistake is when parts of two chromosomes break off and switch with each other. This is called a translocation. It can result in a fusion gene.

Ewing sarcoma is characterized by the fusion of the *EWS* gene (*EWSR1*) on chromosome 22q12 with various members of the *ETS* gene family (*FLI1, ERG, ETV1, ETV4,* and *FEV*). A translocation changes 22q12 to t(11;22). Almost everyone with Ewing sarcoma will have 1 of 4 possible t(11;22) translocations. This is not inherited from your parents, but happens for some other reason. This is called a somatic mutation.

MSI-H/dMMR mutation

Microsatellites are short, repeated strings of DNA. When errors or defects occur, they are fixed. Some cancers prevent these errors from being fixed. This is called microsatellite instability (MSI). When cancer cells have more than a normal number of microsatellites, it is called MSI-H (microsatellite instability-high). Mismatch repair (MMR) helps fix mutations in certain genes. When MMR is lacking or deficient (dMMR), it may lead to cancer.

TMB-H mutations

A tumor with 10 or more mutations is referred to as tumor mutation burden-high (TMB-H).

IDH1 mutation

A sample of your tumor or blood may be used to see if the cancer cells have any specific DNA mutations. Some mutations such as *IDH1* mutations can be targeted with specific therapies. This is a different type of DNA testing than the genetic testing for mutations you may have inherited from your parents. In tumor mutation testing, only the tumor is tested and not the rest of your body. Ivosidenib (Tibsovo®) is for those with chondrosarcoma who are susceptible to *IDH1* mutations.

Cancer stages

A cancer stage is a way to describe the extent of the cancer at the time you are first diagnosed. The American Joint Committee on Cancer (AJCC) created this to determine how much cancer is in your body, where it is located, and what subtype you have. This is called staging. Staging is needed to make treatment decisions. Once treatment starts, staging does not change.

There are other staging systems. Doctors may explain your cancer stage in different ways than described next.

TNM scores

The tumor, node, metastasis (TNM) system is used to stage most bone cancers. In this system, the letters T, N, and M describe different areas of cancer growth. Based on imaging and biopsy results, your doctor will assign a score or number to each letter. The higher the number, the larger the tumor or the more the cancer has spread to lymph nodes or other organs. These scores will be combined to assign the cancer a stage. A TNM example might look like this: T1N0M0 or T1, N0, M0.

- **T (tumor)** - Size of the main (primary) tumor
- **N (node)** - If cancer has spread to nearby (regional) lymph nodes
- **M (metastasis)** - If cancer has spread (metastasized) to distant parts of the body

Cancer staging is often done twice.

- **Clinical stage (c)** is the rating given before any treatment. It is based on a physical exam, biopsy, and imaging tests.
- **Pathologic stage (p)** or surgical stage is determined by examining tissue removed during surgery.

T = Tumor

The primary tumor size is measured in centimeters (cm). A large pea is 1 cm. A golf ball is 4 cm. A baseball is 7 cm. A grapefruit is 15 cm. Tumors are staged based on location.

Bones relating to limbs, torso, skull, and face

The appendicular skeleton is composed of 126 bones of the upper limbs, the lower limbs, the shoulder girdle, and the pelvic girdle. The shoulder girdle is a set of bones that connects the arm to the body. The pelvic girdle is a set of bones that connects the leg to the body.

Staging for tumors found in the appendicular skeleton, torso, skull, and face are described next.

- **TX** Primary tumor cannot be assessed
- **T0** No evidence of primary tumor
- **T1** Tumor is 8 cm or smaller
- **T2** Tumor is larger than 8 cm
- **T3** More than 1 tumor in the primary bone site

Appendicular skeleton

The appendicular skeleton includes the shoulder girdle, the upper limbs, the pelvic girdle, and the lower limbs. The axial skeleton includes the skull, rib cage, and spine.

Reproduced with permission by Cancer Research UK / Wikimedia Commons.

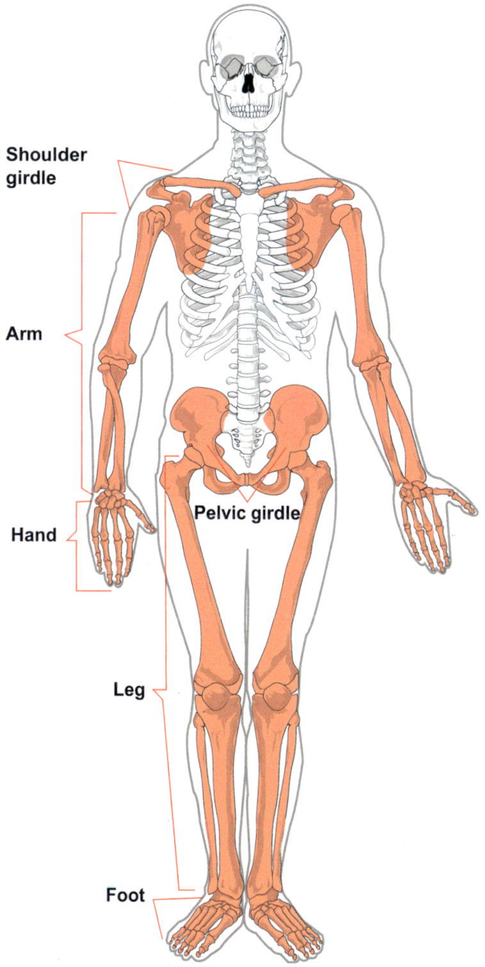

Spine

Staging for tumors found in the bones of the spine (vertebra) are described next.

- **TX** Primary tumor cannot be assessed
- **T0** No evidence of primary tumor
- **T1** Tumor confined to 1 vertebra or 2 adjacent vertebra
- **T2** Tumor confined to 3 adjacent vertebra
- **T3** Tumor confined to 4 or more adjacent vertebra, or any vertebra not next to one another
- **T4** Tumor has grown into spinal canal or large (great) vessels

The spine

The spinal or vertebral column includes a flexible column of bones called vertebrae. The spine includes the sacrum and tailbone (coccyx). There are 24 bones in the flexible spine: 7 cervical (neck), 12 thoracic (upper back), and 5 lumbar (lower back).

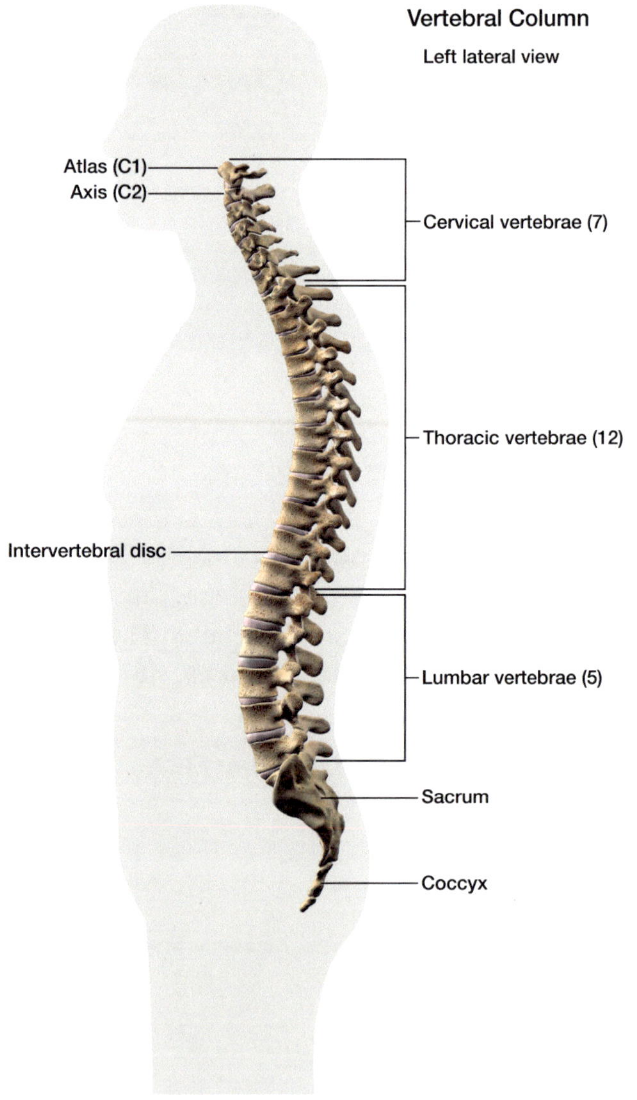

Pelvis

Staging for tumors found in the pelvis are described next.

- **TX** Primary tumor cannot be assessed
- **T0** No evidence of primary tumor
- **T1** Tumor confined to 1 pelvic segment and has not grown outside the bone
  - **T1a** Tumor is 8 cm or less
  - **T1b** Tumor larger than 8 cm
- **T2** Tumor confined to 1 pelvic segment but has grown outside the bone or 2 segments that have not grown outside the bone
  - **T2a** Tumor is 8 cm or less
  - **T2b** Tumor larger than 8 cm
- **T3** Tumor spanning two pelvic segments but has grown outside the bone
  - **T3a** Tumor is 8 cm or less
  - **T3b** Tumor larger than 8 cm
- **T4** Tumor spans 3 pelvic segments or crosses the sacroiliac joint (SIJ)
  - **T4a** Tumor involves sacroiliac joint and extends into the spine
  - **T4b** Tumor has grown into major blood vessels

The pelvis

The pelvis is a basin-shaped structure that supports the spinal column and protects the abdominal organs.

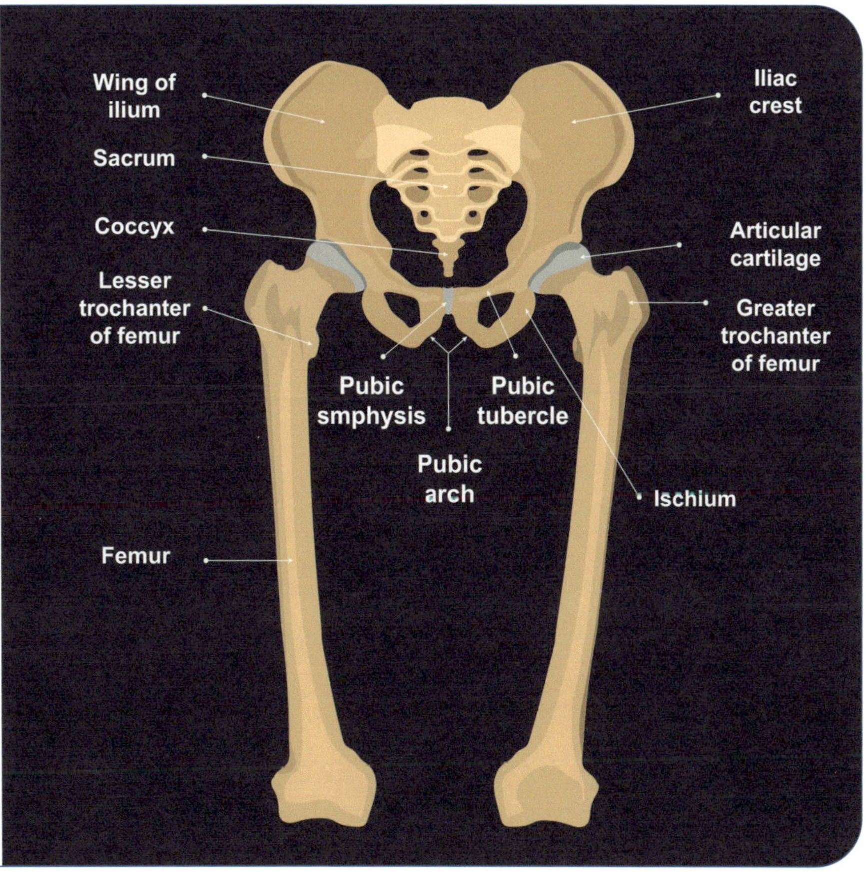

N = Node

There are hundreds of lymph nodes throughout your body. They work as filters to help fight infection and remove harmful things from your body. Regional lymph nodes are those located near tumor. Cancer in the lymph nodes is called nodal disease and is rare in bone cancer.

- **NX** means it cannot be determined
- **N0** means no cancer is found in regional lymph nodes
- **N1** means cancer is found in the regional lymph nodes

M = Metastatic

Cancer that has spread to distant parts of the body is shown as M1. Common sites for metastasis include the lung and bone.

- **M0** means no distant metastasis
- **M1** means distant metastasis is found
    - **M1a** means metastasis in lung
    - **M1b** means metastasis in bone or other distant sites

Grade

Another factor used in staging is the cancer grade. Grade describes how abnormal the tumor cells look under a microscope (histology). Higher-grade cancers tend to grow and spread faster than lower-grade cancers. GX means the grade can't be determined, followed by G1, G2, and G3. Well differentiated (G1) means the cancer cells look like normal cells. Poorly differentiated (G3) means the cancer cells look very different compared to normal cells.

- **GX** Grade cannot be determined
- **G1** Well differentiated – low grade
- **G2** Moderately differentiated – high grade
- **G3** Poorly differentiated – high grade

Numbered stages

Number stages range from stage 1 to stage 4, with 4 being the most advanced. These stages are written as stage I, stage II, stage III, and stage IV. Not all bone cancers are describe this way. See Guide 2.

Guide 2
Bone cancer stages

Stage 1	**Stage 1A**	• T1, N0, M0, G1 or GX
	Stage 1B	• T2, N0, M0, G1 or GX • T3, N0, M0, G1 or GX
Stage 2	**Stage 2A**	• T1, N0, M0, G2 or G3
	Stage 2B	• T2, N0, M0, G2 or G3
Stage 3	**Stage 3**	• T3, N0, M0, G2 or G3
Stage 4	**Stage 4A**	• Any T, N0, M1a, Any G
	Stage 4B	• Any T, N1, Any M, Any G • Any T, Any N, M1b, Any G

Review

- Tests are used to plan treatment and check how well treatment is working.
- Online portals are a great way to access your test results.
- Bone cancer survivors are at risk for fertility issues. Those who want to have children in the future should be referred to a fertility specialist before starting treatment to discuss the options.
- Blood, imaging, and tissue tests check for signs of disease.
- A sample from a biopsy of your tumor might be tested to look for biomarkers or proteins.
- Your health care provider might refer you for genetic testing to learn more about your cancer.
- A cancer stage is a way to describe the extent of the cancer at the time you are first diagnosed.

Fertility issues should be discussed with your doctor before starting chemotherapy.

3 Treating bone cancer

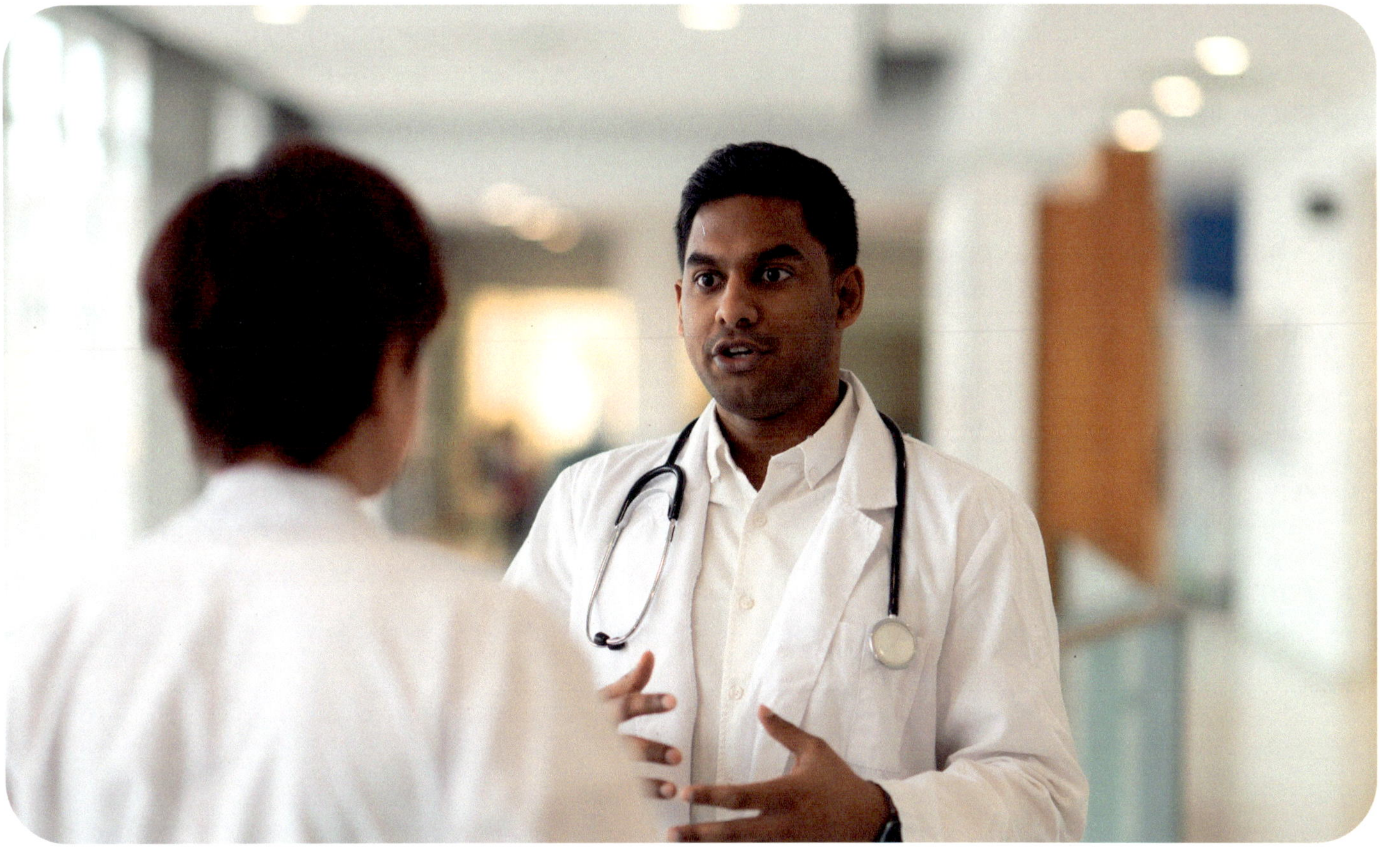

Treatment for bone cancer is based on the type, size, and location of the tumor. This chapter presents an overview of the types of treatment and what to expect. Not everyone will receive the same treatment.

Multidisciplinary team

Treating bone cancer takes a team approach. Treatment decisions should involve a multidisciplinary team (MDT) or a team of doctors from different fields of medicine who have knowledge (expertise) and experience with your type of cancer. This is important. Ask who will coordinate your care.

The MDT should meet on a regular basis and should include the following:

- An orthopedic oncologist specializes in the diagnosis and treatment of bone and soft tissue tumors. They treat any area of the body except the neck and skull and inside the chest and abdomen.
- A bone pathologist interprets the cells and tissues removed during a biopsy or surgery.
- A medical/pediatric oncologist treats cancer using systemic (drug) therapy.
- A radiation oncologist prescribes and plans radiation therapy to treat cancer.
- A musculoskeletal radiologist interprets the results of x-rays and other imaging tests.

Depending on your type of care, the team might include:

- A thoracic surgeon who performs operations within the chest
- A plastic surgeon who performs operations to improve function or reconstruct missing areas
- An interventional radiologist who performs needle biopsies, ablation therapies, and embolizations, and places ports for treatment
- A physiatrist, a medical doctor who specializes in physical movement and rehabilitation
- A vascular surgeon who specializes in procedures involving arteries, veins, and lymph circulation
- A general surgeon who has specialized knowledge and experience related to the diagnosis, preoperative, operative, and postoperative care for the whole patient
- A neurosurgeon who specializes in surgery on the nervous system, especially the brain and spinal cord
- An orthopedic surgeon who focuses on the body's musculoskeletal system, which includes bones, joints, muscles, ligaments, tendons, and nerves
- An orthopedic spine surgeon who specializes in the diagnosis and treatment of spinal diseases and conditions

Some members of your care team will be with you throughout cancer treatment, while others will only be there for parts of it. Get to know your care team and let them get to know you.

Keep a list of names and contact information for each member of your team. This will make it easier for you and anyone involved in your care to know whom to contact with questions or concerns.

You know your body better than anyone. Help other team members understand:

- How you feel
- What you need
- What is working and what is not

Order of treatments

Most people with bone cancer will receive more than one type of treatment. Below is an overview of the order of treatments and what they do.

- **Neoadjuvant (before) treatment** is given to shrink the tumor before primary treatment (surgery). This might change an unresectable tumor into a resectable tumor. Neoadjuvant therapy is often chemotherapy, but might be radiation therapy.
- **Primary treatment** is the main treatment given to rid the body of cancer. Surgery is often the main treatment for many types of bone cancer.
- **Adjuvant (after) treatment** is given after primary treatment to rid the body of any cancer cells left behind from surgery. It is also used when the risk of cancer returning (recurrence) is felt to be high. Adjuvant therapy is often systemic therapy, but might be radiation therapy.
- **First-line treatment** is the first set of systemic (drug) treatment given.
- **Second-line treatment** is the next set of treatment given if cancer progresses during or after systemic therapy.

Surgery

Surgery is an operation or procedure to remove cancer from the body. The type of surgery you receive depends on size, location, and number of tumor(s).

Surgery can be used to:

- Remove all of the tumor
- Relieve pain or discomfort

The goal of surgery is to remove all of the cancer. To do so, the tumor is removed along with some normal-looking tissue around its edge called the surgical margin. A clear or negative margin (R0) is when no cancerous cells are found in the tissue around the edge of the tumor. In an R1 positive margin, the surgeon removes all of the visible tumor, but the microscopic margins are still positive for tumor cells. In an R2 positive margin, the surgeon does not or is unable to remove all of the visible tumor.

A tumor that can be removed completely with surgery is called resectable. Not all tumors are resectable. You might receive treatment to shrink a tumor or the amount of cancer before surgery. This is called preoperative or neoadjuvant treatment. Treatment after surgery might be referred to as postoperative or adjuvant.

When preparing for surgery, seek care or ask for a referral to a hospital or cancer center that has experience in treating your type of bone cancer. It is important to find an experienced surgeon who has performed this type of procedure many times with good results.

Limb-sparing resection

For bone cancer in the limbs, the goal of surgery, whenever possible, is to preserve or maintain limb function. This is called limb-sparing surgery. Rehabilitation, such as physical and occupational therapy, will likely be part of a limb-sparing treatment plan. This may include occupational therapy to help with daily life skills or physical therapy to help your body move and function. A physiatrist is a medical doctor who specializes in rehabilitation.

Amputation

Amputation is the removal of a limb or other body part. A surgeon who is an expert in your type of bone cancer should be consulted before amputation. One type of amputation is a rotationplasty. In a rotationplasty, the bottom of the femur, the knee, and the top of the tibia are removed. The lower leg is then rotated and attached to the femur.

Rehabilitation, such as physical and occupational therapy, will be part of any amputation. Seek a peer support group to connect with others who have experienced the loss of a limb. This will aid in your recovery and help you to maintain an active lifestyle. A physiatrist is a medical doctor who specializes in rehabilitation.

Palliative surgery

Surgery to ease pain or discomfort is called palliative surgery. It might be used to remove metastases that are causing pain. Surgery to remove a metastasis is called a metastasectomy. This is different from a mastectomy which is surgery to remove the breast. Palliative surgery is sometimes offered to fix a broken bone or help prevent a cancerous bone from breaking.

Systemic therapy

Systemic therapy works throughout the body. It includes chemotherapy, targeted therapy, and immunotherapy. Each works differently to shrink the tumor and/or prevent recurrence.

Systemic therapies that might be used include:

- Chemotherapy – attacks rapidly dividing cells in the body
- Targeted therapy – focuses on a specific or unique feature of cancer cells
- Immunotherapy – uses your body's natural defenses to find and destroy cancer cells

Chemotherapy

Chemotherapy kills fast-growing cells throughout the body, including cancer cells and normal cells. All chemotherapies affect the instructions (genes) that tell cancer cells how and when to grow and divide.

Targeted therapy

Targeted therapy focuses on specific or unique features of cancer cells. Targeted therapies seek out how cancer cells grow, divide, and move in the body. These drugs stop the action of molecules that help cancer cells grow and/or survive. Some targeted therapy drugs block the chemical signals that tell cancer cells to grow. Other targeted therapy drugs block signals that cause new blood vessels to form. Others target hormones.

Immunotherapy

Immunotherapy is a targeted therapy that increases the activity of your immune system. By doing so, it improves your body's ability to find and destroy cancer cells. Immunotherapy can be given alone or with other types of treatment. Pembrolizumab (Keytruda®) might be used to treat MSI-H/dMMR tumors. Interferon alfa-2b might be used in some cases to treat giant cell tumor of the bone (GCTB).

Warnings!

You might be asked to stop taking or avoid certain herbal supplements when on a systemic therapy. Some supplements can affect the ability of a drug to do its job. This is called a drug interaction. It is critical to speak with your care team about any supplements you may be taking.

Some examples include:

- Turmeric
- Gingko biloba
- Green tea extract
- St. John's Wort

Even certain medicines can affect the ability of a drug to do its job. Antacids, heart medicine, and antidepressants are just some of the medicines that might interact with a targeted therapy. This is why it is important to tell your doctor about any medications, vitamins, over-the-counter (OTC) drugs, herbals, or supplements you are taking. Bring a list with you to every visit.

Radiation therapy

Radiation therapy (RT) uses high-energy radiation from x-rays, protons, gamma rays, and other sources to kill cancer cells and shrink tumors. Radiation therapy can be given alone, as well as before or after surgery to treat or slow the growth of cancer. Sometimes, radiation is given with chemotherapy. Sometimes, it is given after surgery to reduce the chance that your cancer will return. It may be used as supportive care or palliative care to help ease pain or discomfort caused by cancer that has metastasized to other bones.

Radiation may be given:

- As the primary (first) treatment
- Before surgery, called neoadjuvant radiation therapy, to shrink the tumor before surgery
- After surgery, called adjuvant radiation treatment, to kill any cancerous cells that remain
- As palliative treatment to reduce pain caused by bone metastases

External beam radiation therapy

External beam radiation therapy (EBRT) uses a machine outside of the body to aim radiation at the tumor(s). There is more than one type EBRT used in the treatment of bone cancer. These allow for safer, higher doses of radiation.

Types of EBRT that may be used to treat your cancer include:

- **Stereotactic body radiation therapy (SBRT)** uses high-energy radiation beams to treat cancers in 5 or fewer treatments.
- **Stereotactic radiosurgery (SRS)** uses special equipment to position the body and give one precise, large dose of radiation.
- **Three-dimensional conformal radiation therapy (3D-CRT**) uses computer software and CT images to aim beams that match the shape of the tumor.
- **Intensity-modulated radiation therapy (IMRT)** uses small beams of different strengths to match the shape of the tumor.
- **Particle beam radiation therapy** uses protons, carbon ions, or other heavy ions to treat bone cancer.

Radiopharmaceuticals

Radiopharmaceuticals contain a radioactive substance that emits radiation. This radioactive substance is different than contrast material used in imaging.

Sm 153-EDTMP

Samarium 153-EDTMP or SM^{153}-EDTMP (Quadramet) is a beta-particle–emitting, bone-seeking radiopharmaceutical. It is injected into a vein and distributed throughout the body, where it is absorbed in areas where cancer has invaded the bone.

Palliative radiation therapy

Radiation therapy used to ease pain or discomfort from bone tumors is called palliative RT. Radiation oncologists deliver this treatment.

Clinical trials

Clinical trials study how safe and helpful tests and treatments are for people. Clinical trials find out how to prevent, diagnose, and treat a disease like cancer. Because of clinical trials, scientists and doctors have found, and are continuing to find, new and effective therapies in the management of cancer.

Clinical trials have 4 phases.

- **Phase I trials** aim to find the safest and best dose of a new drug. Another aim is to find the best way to give the drug with the fewest side effects.
- **Phase II trials** assess if a drug works for a specific type of cancer.
- **Phase III trials** formally and scientifically compare a new drug to a standard treatment.
- **Phase IV trials** evaluate a drug's longer term safety and treatment results after it has been approved.

To join a clinical trial, you must meet the conditions of the study. Patients in a clinical trial often are alike in terms of their cancer and general health. This helps to ensure that any change is from the treatment and not because of differences between patients.

If you decide to join a clinical trial, you will need to review and sign a paper called an informed consent form. This form describes the study in detail, including the risks and benefits. Even after you sign a consent form, you can stop taking part in a clinical trial at any time.

Finding a clinical trial

Enrollment in a clinical trial is encouraged when it is the best option for you.

- To find clinical trials online at NCCN Member Institutions, go to NCCN.org/clinical_trials/member_institutions.aspx
- To search the National Institutes of Health (NIH) database for clinical trials in the United States and around the world, go to ClinicalTrials.gov
- To find clinical trials supported by the National Cancer Institute (NCI), go to cancer.gov/about-cancer/treatment/clinical-trials/search

Ask your cancer team for help finding a clinical trial. You may also get help from NCI's Cancer Information Service (CIS). Call 1.800.4.CANCER (1.800.422.6237) or go to cancer.gov/contact

Ask your treatment team if there is an open clinical trial that you can join. There may be clinical trials where you're getting treatment or at other treatment centers nearby. Discuss the risks and benefits of joining a clinical trial with your care team. Together, decide if a clinical trial is right for you.

Other treatments

Ablation

Ablation uses extreme cold or extreme heat to destroy cancer cells. It can destroy small tumors with little harm to nearby tissue.

There are 2 types of thermal ablation used to destroy cancer cells:

- Cryotherapy or cryosurgery
- Radiofrequency ablation (RFA)

Both types of ablation use a special needle, called a probe, which is inserted into the tumor. With cryotherapy, a medical gas is passed through the probe to cause below-freezing temperatures. This freezes the tumor to destroy it. With RFA, the probe emits radio waves to heat the tumor and destroy it. The probe can be guided into place with a CT scan, ultrasound, or other imaging tests. The probe will be removed when treatment is done.

Embolization

Embolization treats tumors by cutting off their blood supply. A catheter will be inserted into an artery and guided to the tumor. Once in place, beads will be inserted to block the blood flow.

With chemoembolization, the beads are coated with chemotherapy. Radioembolization uses small radioactive beads.

Supportive care

Supportive care is health care that relieves symptoms caused by cancer or its treatment and improves quality of life. It might include pain relief (palliative care), emotional or spiritual support, financial aid, or family counseling. Supportive care is given during all cancer stages. Tell your care team how you are feeling and about any side effects. Best supportive care is used with other treatments to improve quality of life. Best supportive care, supportive care, and palliative care are often used interchangeably.

Review

- Treatment decisions should involve a multidisciplinary team (MDT) or a team of doctors from different fields of medicine who have knowledge (expertise) and experience with your type of cancer.
- Surgery to remove a metastasis is called a metastasectomy. This is different from a mastectomy, which is surgery to remove the breast.
- Systemic therapy works throughout the body. It includes chemotherapy, targeted therapy, and immunotherapy.
- Radiation therapy (RT) uses high-energy radiation from x-rays, protons, gamma rays, and other sources to kill cancer cells and shrink tumors.
- Ablation uses extreme cold or extreme heat to destroy cancer cells.
- Embolization treats tumors by cutting off their blood supply.
- Supportive care is health care that relieves symptoms caused by cancer or its treatment and improves quality of life.

Tell your doctor about any medications, vitamins, over-the-counter drugs, herbals, or supplements you are taking.

4 Chondrosarcoma

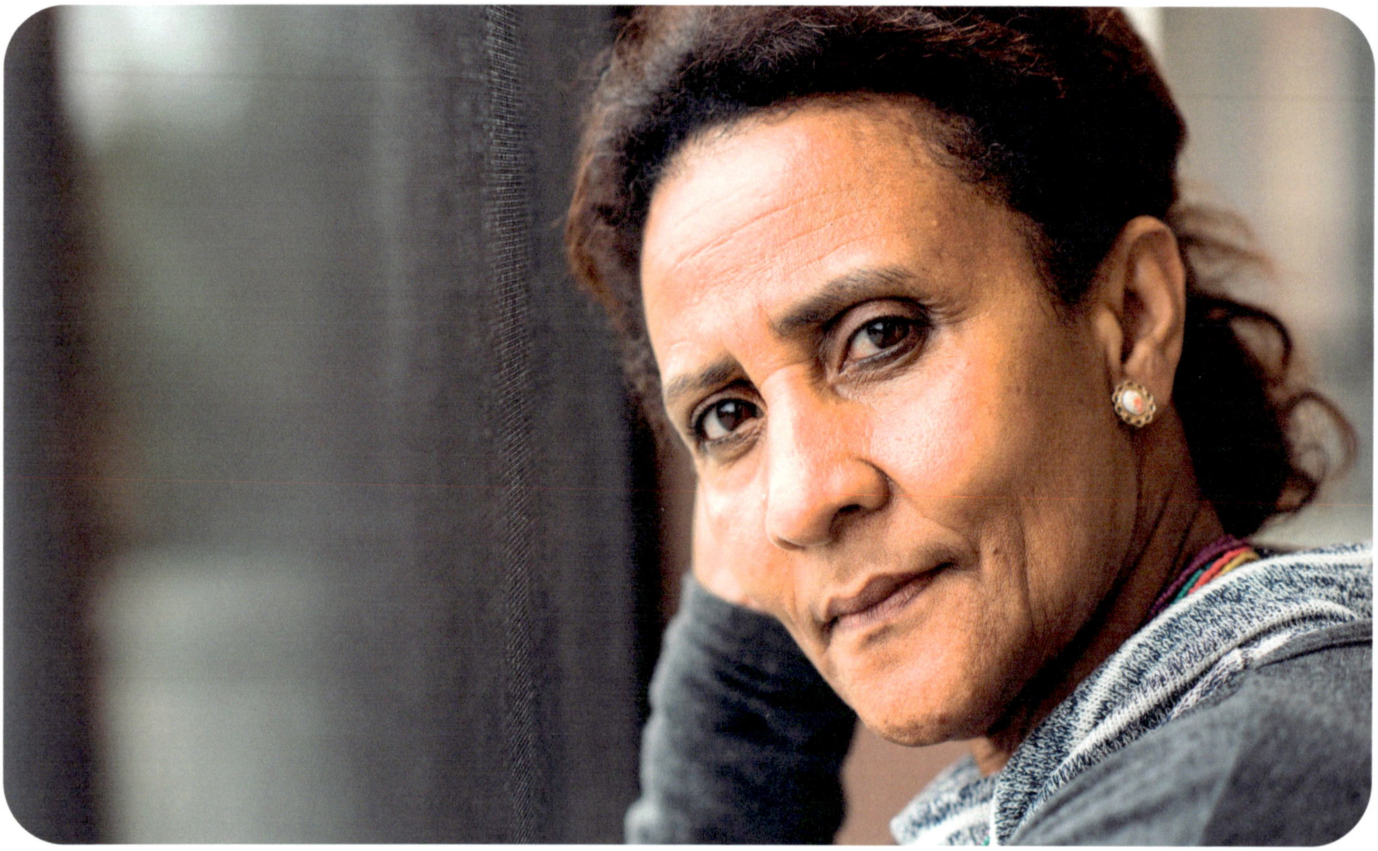

Chondrosarcoma starts in the cells that form cartilage. Treatment is usually surgery to remove the tumor or radiation therapy. Together, you and your doctor will choose a treatment plan that is best for you.

Overview

Chondrosarcoma starts in the cells that form cartilage. It is most commonly found in the thigh bone (femur), arm (humerus), or pelvis. Treatment is based on the grade of the tumor and if it can be removed with surgery.

A tumor that can be removed with surgery is called resectable. An unresectable tumor cannot be removed with surgery. Surgery to remove all of the tumor is called wide excision.

Treatment is grouped as follows:

- Low grade and intracompartmental
- High grade (grade 2 or 3), clear cell, or extracompartmental
- Metastatic disease at initial diagnosis
- For poorly differentiated or dedifferentiated, some doctors may treat as osteosarcoma
- For mesenchymal, some doctors may treat as Ewing sarcoma

Treatment options will be based on your wishes and your doctor's recommendations. See Guide 3.

Guide 3
Treatment options: Chondrosarcoma

Low grade and intracompartmental	• Intralesional surgery (curettage) to remove part of the tumor (not an option for pelvic tumors). Might be followed by more surgery. • If resectable, surgery to remove all of the tumor (wide excision). • If unresectable, consider radiation therapy (RT).	→ If cancer returns, the options are: • If resectable, wide excision. If surgery does not remove all of the cancer, then you might have more surgery or RT. • If unresectable, consider RT.
High grade, clear cell, or extracompartmental	• If resectable, surgery to remove all of the tumor (wide excision). • If borderline resectable or unresectable, consider radiation therapy (RT).	

Treatment

Low grade and intracompartmental

A low-grade and intracompartmental tumor is still within the bone. It has not grown through the bone wall or spread to any other part of the body.

Depending on the location of the tumor, treatment options include:

- Intralesional surgery (curettage) to remove part of the tumor (not an option for pelvic tumors). Might be followed by more surgery.
- If resectable, surgery to remove all of the tumor (wide excision)
- If unresectable, consider radiation therapy

Monitoring

After treatment you will be monitored for recurrence. When cancer returns, it is called recurrence.

You will have the following tests:

- Physical exam
- X-rays of primary site and/or MRI or CT (both with contrast) as needed every 6 to 12 months for 2 years, then yearly
- Chest imaging every 6 to 12 months for 2 years, then yearly

High grade, clear cell, or extracompartmental

Tumors that are high grade, clear cell, or extracompartmental follow the treatment outlined below. A tumor that is high grade (grade 2 or 3) looks very abnormal under a microscope. Clear cell is a type of chondrosarcoma. An extracompartmental bone cancer has grown through the bone wall and out of the area where it started.

Treatment options include:

- If resectable, surgery to remove all of the tumor (wide excision)
- If borderline resectable or unresectable, consider radiation therapy

Monitoring

After treatment you will be monitored for signs that cancer has returned.

You will have the following tests:

- Physical exam
- X-rays of primary site and/or MRI or CT (both with contrast) as needed
- Chest imaging every 3 to 6 months, may include chest CT at least every 6 months for 5 years, then every year for at least 10 years
- Re-assess function every follow-up visit

Recurrence

Cancer that has returned after a disease-free period is called recurrence.

If cancer returns at or near the same place, then the treatment options are:

- If resectable, surgery to remove all of the tumor (wide excision). If surgery does not remove all of the cancer, then you might have more surgery or radiation therapy.
- If unresectable, consider radiation therapy

Metastatic disease

Treatment for metastatic chondrosarcoma is based on if there are a few metastases called oligometastases or if the cancer is widespread. Treatment focuses on reducing the number of metastases or amount of cancer. See Guide 4.

Oligometastases

In oligometastases, there are a limited number of metastases. If possible, you will have surgery to remove all of the metastases. Radiation therapy is an option for unresectable metastases. A clinical trial is also an option.

Widespread disease

Treatment options for widespread disease might include:

- Radiation therapy, surgery, and/or ablation therapies
- Dasatinib or pazopanib
- Clinical trial

Before starting systemic therapy, tumor mutation burden (TMB) testing might be done. Not everyone with metastatic chondrosarcoma is able to have surgery or systemic therapy. Ivosidenib (Tibsovo®) would be an option for these patients who have susceptible *IDH1* mutations.

Guide 4
Treatment options: Metastatic chondrosarcoma

Oligometastases	• Surgery to remove all metastases if possible • Consider radiation therapy for unresectable metastases • Consider clinical trial
Widespread disease	• Consider radiation therapy, surgery, and/or ablation therapies for sites causing symptoms • Consider tumor mutation burden (TMB) testing • Consider dasatinib (Sprycel™) or pazopanib (Votrient) • Consider clinical trial • Ivosidenib (Tibsovo®) might be an option for those who have susceptible *IDH1* mutations

Review

- Chondrosarcoma starts in the cells that form cartilage.
- Treatment is based on the grade of the tumor and if it can be removed with surgery.
- A tumor that can be removed with surgery is called resectable.
- An unresectable tumor cannot be removed with surgery. Unresectable tumors are often treated with radiation therapy (RT).
- Surgery to remove all of a tumor is called wide excision.
- A clinical trial is an option for metastatic chondrosarcoma.
- The goal of treatment for metastatic chondrosarcoma is to reduce the number of metastases or the amount of cancer in the body.

Get to know your care team and let them get to know you.

5 Chordoma

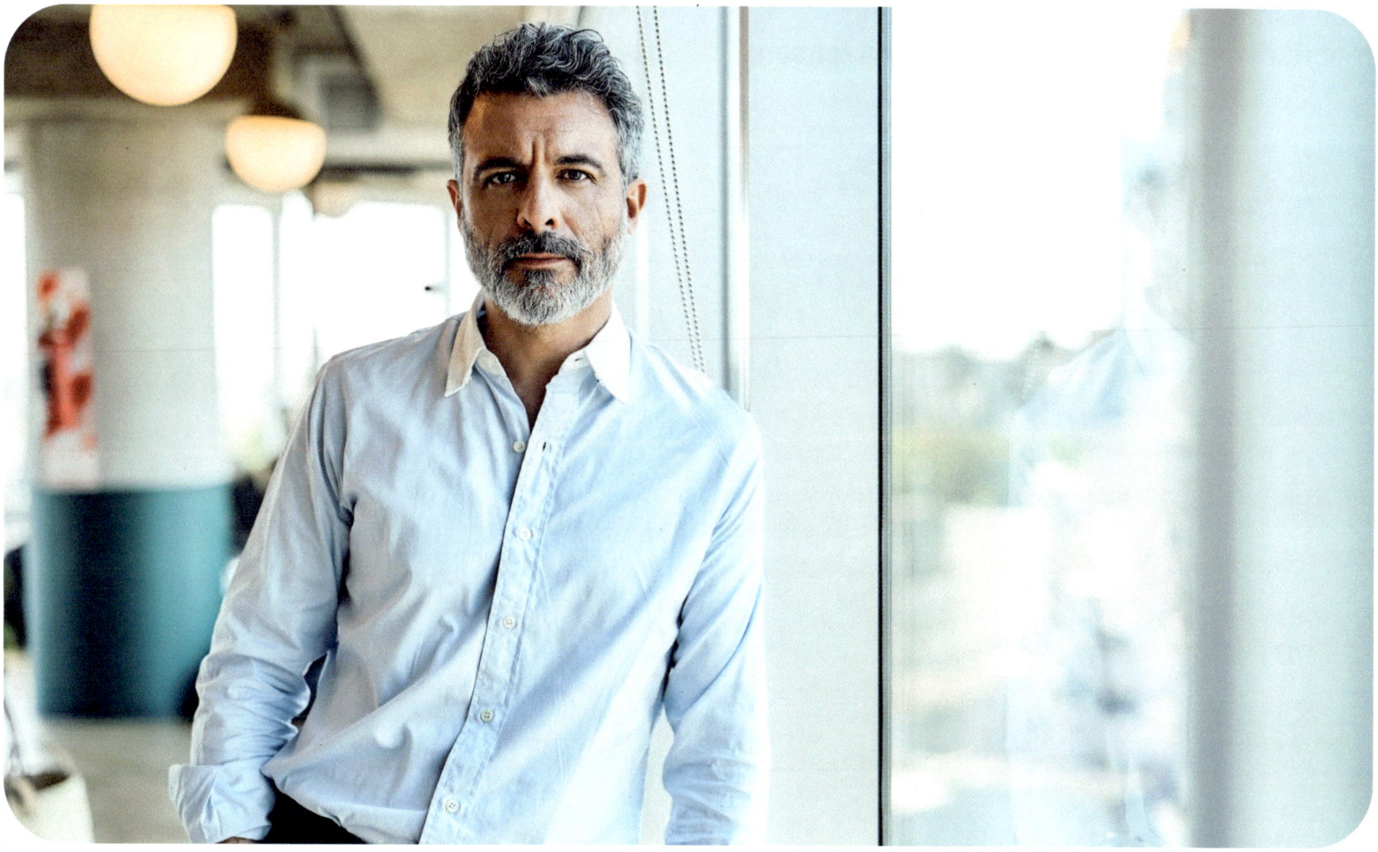

Chordoma is a slow-growing sarcoma that usually starts in the lower spinal column or at the base of the skull. It often grows into the soft tissue around the bone making it difficult to treat. Treatment options include surgery or radiation therapy. Together, you and your doctor will choose a treatment plan that is best for you.

Overview

Chordomas are a type of cancerous tumor that can occur anywhere along the spine, from the base of the skull to the tailbone. Tumors grow slowly, gradually invading nearby bone and soft tissue.

Tumors often involve critical structures such as the brainstem, spinal cord, and important nerves and arteries. For this reason, chordomas are difficult to treat. They can also come back, or recur, after treatment — usually in the same place as the first tumor. This is called a local recurrence. In about 2 out of 5 people, the tumor eventually spreads, or metastasizes, to other parts of the body.

This chapter is for conventional or chondroid types of chordomas.

For those with poorly differentiated or dedifferentiated chordoma, please see the *NCCN Guidelines for Patients: Soft Tissue Sarcoma* at NCCN.org/patientguidelines.

Testing

Those with chordoma should be evaluated and treated by a multidisciplinary team of doctors who are experts in the management of chordoma. Before starting treatment, you will have tests found in Guide 5.

Guide 5 **Testing for chordoma**
Those with chordoma should be evaluated and treated by a multidisciplinary team with expertise in the management of chordoma
Medical history and physical exam
Imaging of primary site that might include x-ray, CT and/or MRI, and screening MRI of spine
Chest/abdominal/pelvic CT with contrast
PET/CT (skull base to mid-thigh)
Consider bone scan

Treatment

Chordomas are treated based on the location of the tumor:

- Tumors in the spine that include the sacrum and coccyx
- Tumors at or in the base of the skull

A tumor that can be removed with surgery is called resectable. An unresectable tumor cannot be removed with surgery and might be treated with radiation therapy (RT). Chordomas often grown outside the bone into surrounding tissue near vital organs, veins, and arteries. Parts of these tissues might also need to be removed and sewn back together. This is called resection. The goal is to remove as much of the tumor as possible.

For all treatment options see Guide 6.

Tumors in spine

For tumors in the spine:

- If a tumor is resectable, RT might be given before, during, or after surgery.
- If a tumor is unresectable, then RT might be an option.

Tumors in skull base

For tumors at or in the base of the skull:

- If a tumor is resectable, RT might be given before, during, or after surgery. A follow-up MRI with contrast will be done to see if RT or another surgery is needed.
- If a tumor is unresectable, then RT might be an option.

Monitoring

After completing treatment, you will be monitored to watch for signs that cancer has returned called recurrence. Monitoring includes a physical exam and imaging tests.

Guide 6
Treatment options: Chordoma recurrence

Local recurrence	• Surgical excision and/or • Radiation therapy and/or • Systemic therapy (see Guide 7)
Metastatic recurrence	• Systemic therapy (see Guide 7) and/or • Surgical excision and/or • Radiation therapy and/or • Best supportive care

Recurrence

When cancer returns, it is called recurrence. Treatment is based on if it the recurrence is local or metastatic. In local recurrence, cancer returns close to where there initial tumor was found. In metastatic recurrence, cancer is found in bones or other parts of the body far from the original site.

Treatment might include surgery, systemic therapy, or radiation therapy. These treatments might be used alone or in combination. Systemic therapy is drug therapy that works throughout the body. Most systemic therapy options for chordoma recurrence are targeted therapies. Best supportive care is given with metastatic recurrence. Best supportive care is treatment to improve quality of life.

For systemic therapy options see Guide 7.

Review

- Chordomas are treated based on the location of the tumor.
- A tumor that can be removed with surgery is called resectable. The goal of surgery is to remove as much of the tumor as possible.
- An unresectable tumor cannot be removed with surgery and might be treated with radiation therapy (RT).
- When cancer returns, it is called recurrence. In local recurrence, cancer returns close to where there initial tumor was found. In metastatic recurrence, cancer is found in bones or other parts of the body far from the original site.
- Best supportive care is treatment to improve quality of life.

Guide 7
Systemic therapy options: Chordoma recurrence

Preferred options	—
Other recommended	• Imatinib • Dasatinib • Sunitinib
Used in some cases	• Imatinib with cisplatin or sirolimus • Erlotinib • Lapatinib for EGFR-positive chordomas • Sorafenib

6
Ewing sarcoma

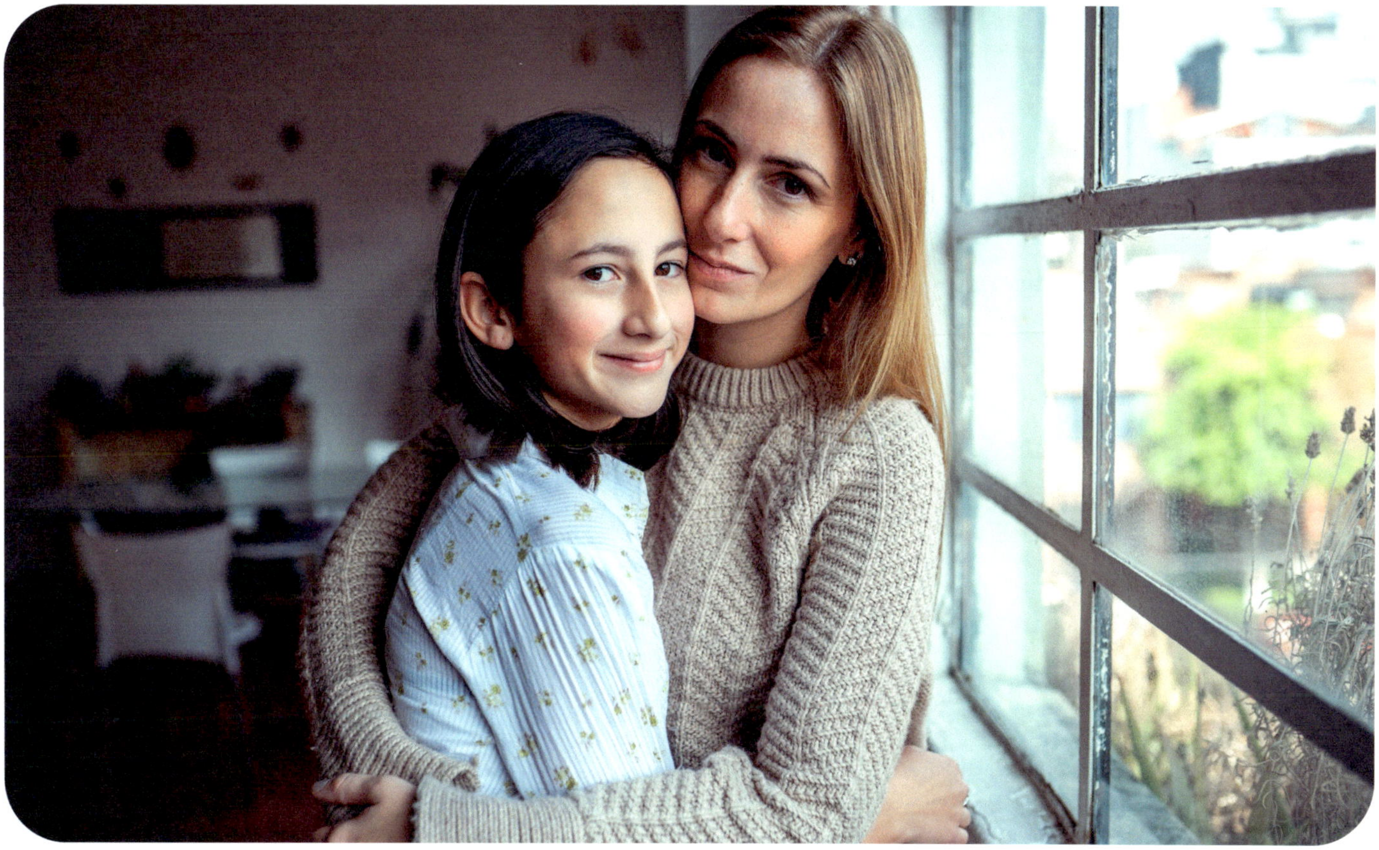

Ewing sarcoma is a group of cancers that start in the bone or soft tissue. Treatment begins with chemotherapy. Together, you and your doctor will choose a treatment plan that is best for you.

Overview

Ewing sarcoma is a cancerous tumor that occurs in bone or soft tissue. Soft tissue includes cartilage or nerves.

There are 2 types of Ewing sarcoma:

- Ewing sarcoma of bone
- Ewing sarcoma of soft tissues

Ewing sarcoma of bone usually occurs in the thigh (femur), pelvis, and bones of the chest. Although, any bone may be affected. When arising in a long bone, the diaphysis is the most common site. Ewing sarcoma can spread to other parts of the body (metastasize), usually to the lungs, to other bones, or to the bone marrow.

Testing

Before starting treatment, you will have tests found in Guide 8.

Guide 8 Testing for Ewing sarcoma
Medical history and physical exam
MRI with or without CT (both with contrast) of primary site
Chest x-ray
PET/CT (head-to-toe) and/or bone scan
Consider bone marrow biopsy and/or screening MRI of spine and pelvis
Cytogenetics and/or molecular testing (may require re-biopsy)
Lactate dehydrogenase (LDH)
Fertility consultation should be considered

Primary treatment

Chemotherapy is the first or primary treatment for all types of Ewing sarcoma. It will include a combination of chemotherapies. This is called multiagent chemotherapy. You will have at least 9 weeks of multiagent first-line chemotherapy. See Guide 9.

Restaging

After primary treatment of first-line chemotherapy, your cancer will be restaged.

Tests to restage your cancer might include:

- Chest CT
- MRI with or with CT (both with contrast) of primary site
- PET/CT (head-to-toe) or bone scan (whichever was done before)

Restaging will determine if the cancer is:

- Stable or improved
- Not responding to treatment or has progressed

Guide 9
First-line chemotherapy options: Ewing sarcoma

Preferred option	• Vincristine, doxorubicin, and cyclophosphamide alternating with ifosfamide and etoposide (VDC/IE). Dactinomycin can be substituted for doxorubicin.
Other recommended	• Vincristine, doxorubicin, and ifosfamide (VAI) • Vincristine, ifosfamide, doxorubicin, and etoposide (VIDE)

Adjuvant treatment

Adjuvant treatment follows primary treatment. This section is for those with stable or improved disease following primary therapy.

Adjuvant treatment might be:

- Surgery to remove the tumor (wide excision). Radiation might be given before surgery.
- Definitive radiation therapy (RT) and chemotherapy
- Amputation in some cases

A definitive treatment is defined as the best treatment after all choices have been considered. Treatment after surgery or amputation is based on if cancer was found in the surgical margin. When cancer is found in the surgical margin, it is called positive or a positive surgical margin. Treatment might be chemotherapy, RT, or a combination of both. See Guide 10.

Guide 10
Adjuvant treatment options: Ewing sarcoma

Stable or improved disease	Wide excision →	If cancer found in surgical margin, the options are: • Continue chemotherapy (see Guide 9) followed by radiation therapy (RT) or • RT and chemotherapy
		If no cancer found in surgical margin, the option is: • Chemotherapy (see Guide 9) and consider RT for pelvic tumors
	Definitive RT and chemotherapy	
	Amputation in some cases →	Followed by chemotherapy, consider RT depending on if cancer found in surgical margin

Monitoring

After completing treatment, you will be monitored to watch for signs that cancer has returned (relapsed). Monitoring includes physical exam and imaging tests. See Guide 11.

Relapse

Cancer that returns after a disease-free period is called relapse. Treatment is chemotherapy with or without radiation therapy. In early relapse, less than 2 years has passed since initial diagnosis. A different chemotherapy will be tried. For late relapse, the same chemotherapy might be tried again.

Guide 11 Monitoring Ewing sarcoma
Physical exam
MRI with or without CT (both with contrast) of primary site
Chest imaging (x-ray or CT) every 2 to 3 months
X-rays of primary site
Complete blood count (CBC) and other blood tests
Increase intervals for physical exam, imaging of primary site and chest after 2 years and annually after 5 years (indefinitely)
Consider PET/CT (head-to-toe) or bone scan

Disease progression

When cancer does not respond or progresses after first-line chemotherapy, then radiation therapy (RT) and/or surgery might be considered to prevent the spread of cancer or to ease pain. If cancer continues to progress or relapses, then options include a second-line chemotherapy or best supportive care. A relapse is the return of cancer. Supportive care is not treatment aimed to cure cancer, but treatment to improve quality of life. For second-line chemotherapy options, see Guide 12.

A preferred treatment option is proven to be more effective.

Guide 12
Second-line chemotherapy options: Ewing sarcoma

Preferred options	• Cyclophosphamide and topotecan. Vincristine might be added. • Irinotecan and temozolomide. Vincristine might be added.
Other recommended	• Cabozantinib • Docetaxel and gemcitabine. Vincristine might be added.
Used in some cases	• Ifosfamide, carboplatin, and etoposide. Vincristine might be added.

Metastatic treatment

Metastatic Ewing sarcoma is cancer found throughout the body. Treatment for an initial diagnosis of metastatic Ewing sarcoma is different than cancer that has spread during or after treatment. This section is for those with metastatic Ewing sarcoma at diagnosis.

Treatment focuses on the primary (main) site and/or the distant metastases. In other words, treatment might include surgery or radiation therapy (RT) of the main site with treatment for the metastatic sites.

Lungs, bone, and bone marrow are the most common sites of metastasis. Often, a lung metastasis is easier to treat than a metastasis found in other sites. Treatment for a lung metastasis might include surgery and/or RT.

For treatment of an initial diagnosis of metastatic Ewing sarcoma, see Guide 13.

Guide 13
Treatment options: Metastatic Ewing sarcoma as initial diagnosis

Local control therapy for main site	Wide excision →	If cancer found in surgical margin, the options are: • Continue chemotherapy (see Guide 14) followed by radiation therapy (RT) or • RT and chemotherapy
		If no cancer found in surgical margin, the option is: • Chemotherapy (see Guide 14) • RT might be considered for close margin
	Definitive RT and chemotherapy (see Guide 14)	
Widely metastatic	• Continuing chemotherapy only with palliative surgery • Palliative RT to symptomatic areas • Other techniques for multiple metastases	

Local control therapy

Treatment that focuses on the primary tumor is called local control therapy.

There are 2 options:

- Surgery to remove the tumor (wide excision). RT might be given before surgery.
- Definitive RT and chemotherapy

A definitive treatment is defined as the best treatment after all choices have been considered. Treatment after surgery is based on if cancer was found in the surgical margin. When cancer is found in the surgical margin, it is called positive. Treatment might be chemotherapy, RT, or a combination of both. If after treatment, a metastasis is found, you might have surgery or RT, or both.

Chemotherapy options can be found in Guide 14.

Widely metastatic

Treatment for widely metastatic disease might include chemotherapy, palliative surgery, or palliative radiation. Other techniques might be used to treat metastases.

Guide 14
Metastatic chemotherapy options: Ewing sarcoma

Preferred options	• Vincristine, doxorubicin, and cyclophosphamide alternating with ifosfamide and etoposide (VDC/IE) • Vincristine, doxorubicin, and ifosfamide (VAI) • Vincristine, ifosfamide, doxorubicin, and etoposide (VIDE) • Vincristine, doxorubicin, and cyclophosphamide (VDC)

* Dactinomycin can be substituted for doxorubicin

Review

- Chemotherapy is the first or primary treatment for all types of Ewing sarcoma.
- After primary treatment, your cancer will be restaged.
- Adjuvant treatment follows primary treatment. Adjuvant treatment is based on how your cancer responded to primary treatment of chemotherapy.
- Metastatic cancer is cancer found throughout the body. Treatment for an initial diagnosis of metastatic Ewing sarcoma is different than cancer that has spread during or after treatment.
- Treatment that focuses on the primary tumor is called local control therapy.
- Treatment for widely metastatic disease might include chemotherapy, palliative surgery, or palliative radiation.

Create a medical binder

A medical binder or notebook is a great way to organize all of your records in one place.

- Make copies of blood tests, imaging results, and reports about your specific type of cancer. It will be helpful when getting a second opinion.
- Choose a binder that meets your needs. Consider a zipper pocket to include a pen, small calendar, and insurance cards.
- Create folders for insurance forms, medical records, and tests results. You can do the same on your computer.
- Use online patient portals to view your test results and other records. Download or print the records to add to your binder.
- Organize your binder in a way that works for you. Add a section for questions and to take notes.
- Bring your medical binder to appointments. You never know when you might need it!

7
Giant cell tumor of the bone

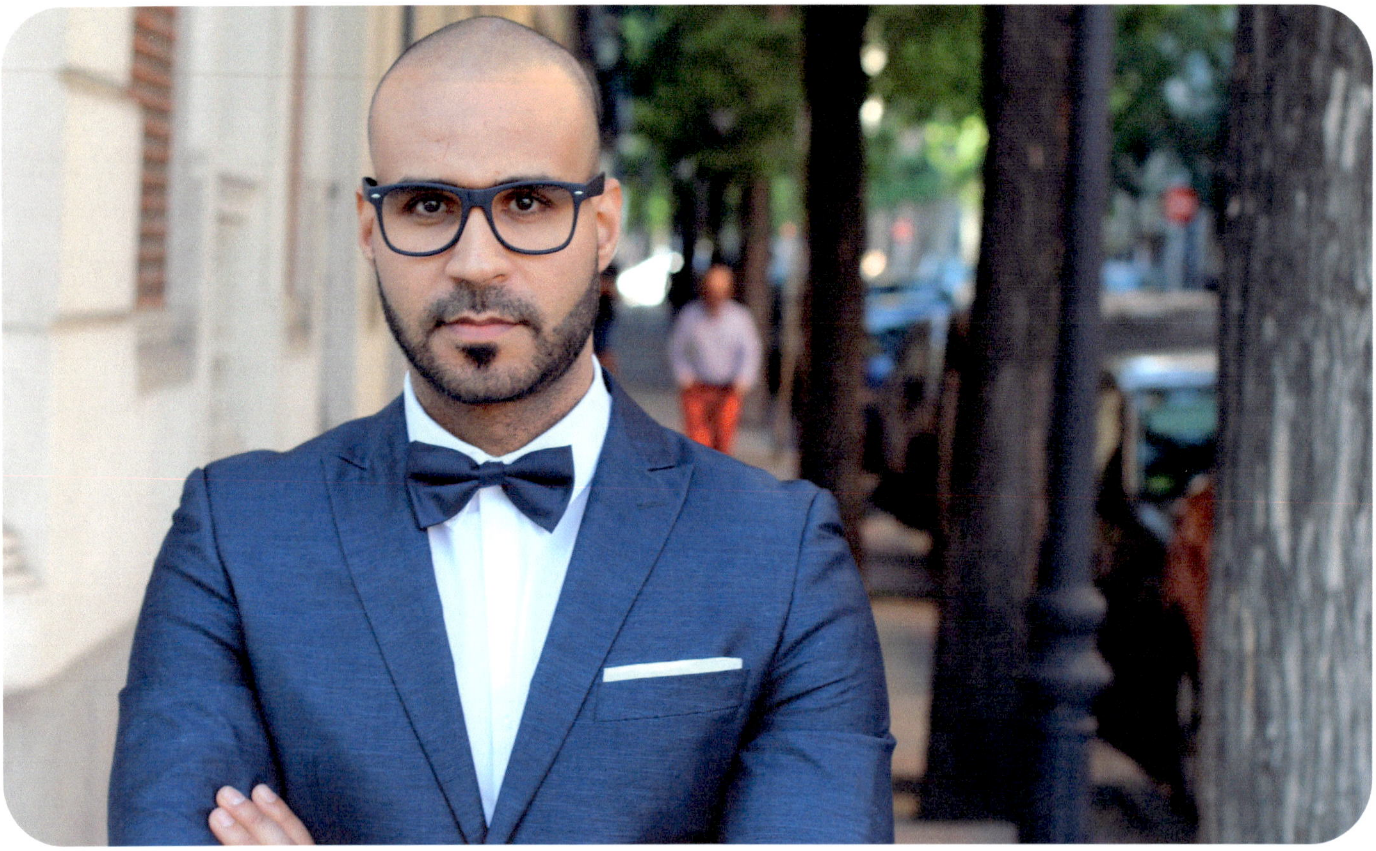

Giant cell tumor of the bone (GCTB) is usually benign (not cancer). However, it is an aggressive, unpredictable disease that tends to return. Treatment is needed to prevent severe bone damage. Together, you and your doctor will choose a treatment plan that is best for you.

Overview

Giant cell tumor of bone (GCTB) is a rare, aggressive non-cancerous tumor. It generally happens in adults between ages 20 and 40 when skeletal bone growth is complete.

When viewed under a microscope, the tumor consists of many very large or "giant" cells.

It is not known what causes a giant cell tumor. GCTB usually develops near a joint at the end of the bone. The knee is the most common location, but can be found in the bones of the arms and the legs. It can also affect the flat bones, such as the breastbone or pelvis.

GCTB has a strong tendency to return to the same location. This is called local recurrence. It may metastasize to the lungs.

When possible, treatment for a giant cell tumor almost always involves surgery to remove the tumor. Treatment aims to prevent damage to the bone near the affected joint.

Giant cell tumor of the bone

Giant cell tumors are often found at the end of the thigh bone (femur).

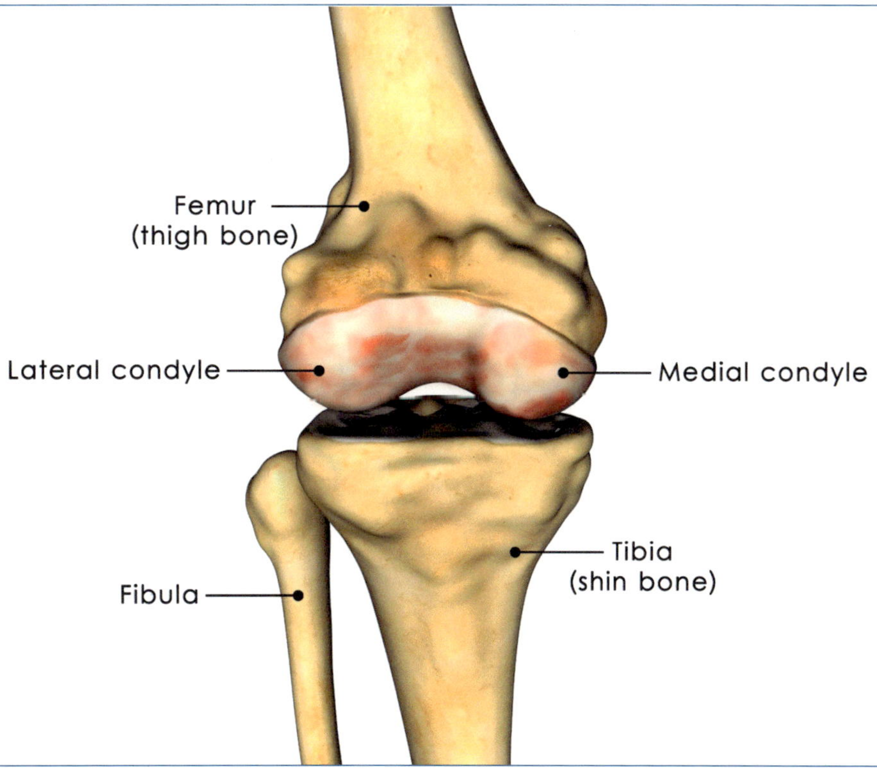

Testing

Before starting treatment, you will have tests to see if the cancer is in one area (localized) or has spread to distant sites (metastasized). See Guide 15.

Localized disease

In localized disease, cancer is confined to one area. Due to the location of the tumor or if you have other more serious health issues, surgery might not be possible. If this is the case, see unresectable treatment options.

Resectable

A resectable tumor can be removed with surgery. When possible, you will have surgery to remove the tumor. At the time of surgery, your surgeon will might use treatment (cautery, chemicals, or heat/cold) to help prevent the return of the tumor.

Unresectable

An unresectable tumor cannot be removed with surgery. Those with an unresectable tumor might include those with a resectable tumor, but who have other more serious health conditions that prevent surgery.

Treatments include:

- Denosumab (preferred) and/or
- Embolization (preferred) and/or
- Interferon alfa-2b (used in some cases) and/or
- Radiation therapy (RT)

There are some risks with RT. Discuss with your doctor which treatment is right for you.

After treatment you will have imaging tests, such as x-rays, CT, and MRI, to check for response. If tests find that the tumor is now resectable, you will have surgery to remove the tumor.

Guide 15 Testing for GCTB
Medical history and physical exam
Imaging of primary site that might include x-ray, CT with contrast, and/or MRI with contrast
Chest imaging
Consider bone scan
Biopsy to confirm diagnosis
If malignant, treat as osteosarcoma

Metastatic disease

In metastatic disease, there is more than one tumor. GCTB may metastasize to the lungs or other bone.

For resectable tumors, you might have surgery to remove:

- Primary tumor
- Metastasis

For unresectable tumors, your doctor will consider the following options:

- Denosumab
- Interferon alfa-2b (used in some cases)
- Radiation therapy
- Observation

Observation is sometimes referred to as watch-and-wait. Ask your doctor what this might mean for you.

Monitoring

After completing treatment, you will be monitored to watch for signs that cancer has returned called recurrence. Monitoring includes physical exam and imaging tests of the surgical site. You will have chest imaging to look for lung metastases. See Guide 16.

Recurrence

GCTB often returns to the same area called local recurrence. There is concern it can spread (metastasize) to the lungs. Treatment is based on if it is a local or metastatic recurrence. For metastatic recurrence, see "Metastatic disease" in this chapter.

Local recurrence

For a resectable tumor, you might have chest CT to see if there are any metastases in the lungs. Denosumab might be given before surgery to remove the primary tumor (wide excision). Both resectable and unresectable treatment will follow "Localized disease" in this chapter.

Guide 16
Monitoring GCTB

Physical exam
Imaging of surgical site that might include x-ray and CT with or without MRI (both with contrast)
Chest imaging every 6 months, then annually thereafter

Review

- Giant cell tumor of the bone (GCTB) consists of many very large or "giant" cells.
- When possible, treatment for a giant cell tumor almost always involves surgery to remove the tumor. Treatment aims to prevent damage to the bone near the affected joint.
- Before starting treatment, you will have tests to see if the cancer is in one area (localized) or has spread to distant sites (metastasized). Treatment will be based on if surgery is possible.
- In metastatic disease, there is more than one tumor. GCTB may metastasize to the lungs or other bone.
- After completing treatment, you will be monitored to watch for signs that cancer has returned called recurrence.
- GTCB often returns to the same area called recurrence. Treatment is based on if it is a local or metastatic recurrence.

8 Osteosarcoma

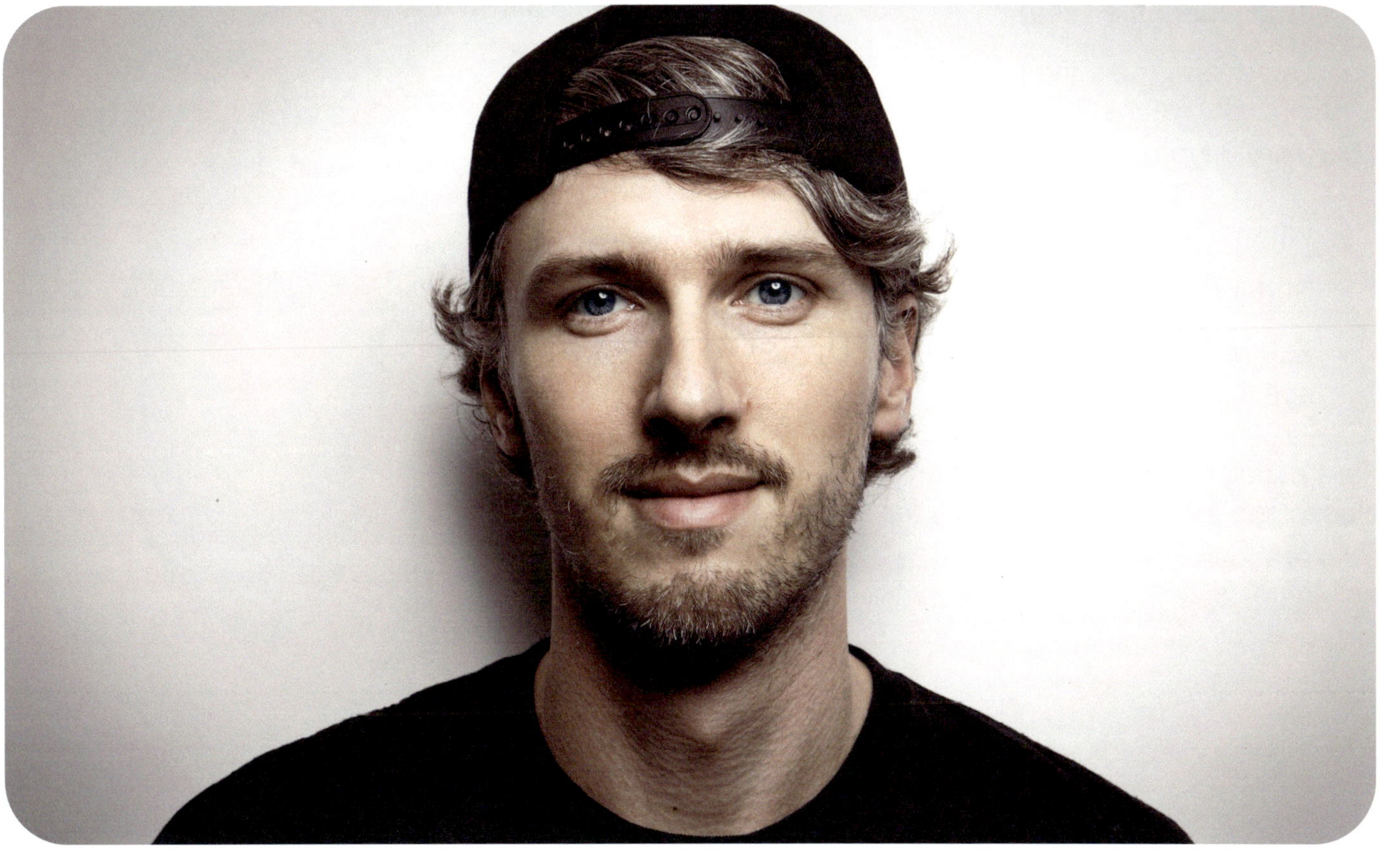

Osteosarcoma is the most common type of bone cancer. It usually occurs in the thigh, upper arm, or shin. Treatment is a combination of therapies. Together, you and your doctor will choose a treatment plan that is best for you.

Overview

Osteosarcoma starts in bone-forming cells called osteoblasts. The cause is not known. In some cases, osteosarcoma runs in families. Osteosarcoma is commonly found in large bones in the area of bone with the fastest growth rate. However, it can occur in any bone.

Osteosarcoma tends to occur in bones of the:

- Shin (near the knee)
- Thigh (near the knee)
- Upper arm (near the shoulder)

There are 3 types of osteosarcoma:

- Intramedullary (inside the bone)
- Surface (on the bone surface)
- Extraskeletal (outside the bone known as soft tissue sarcoma)

For treating extraskeletal osteosarcomas, please see the *NCCN Guidelines for Patients: Soft Tissue Sarcoma* at NCCN.org/patientguidelines.

Testing

Before starting treatment, you will have the tests found in Guide 17.

Guide 17 Testing for osteosarcoma
Medical history and physical exam
MRI with or without CT (both with contrast) of primary site
Chest imaging including chest CT
PET/CT (head-to-toe) and/or bone scan
MRI or CT (both with contrast) of skeletal metastatic sites
Lactate dehydrogenase (LDH)
Alkaline phosphatase (ALP)
Fertility consultation should be considered
Consider personal and family history for genetic consultation and testing

Systemic therapy

Treatment for osteosarcoma is a combination of therapies. Chemotherapy and other systemic therapies are often part of treatment for osteosarcoma. First-line chemotherapies are those tried first. Second-line systemic therapy options are used when disease progresses or does not respond to first-line options.

For possible first-line chemotherapies, see Guide 18.

For possible second-line systemic therapies, see Guide 19.

Guide 18
First-line chemotherapy options: Osteosarcoma

Preferred options	• Cisplatin and doxorubicin • High-dose methotrexate, cisplatin, and doxorubicin (MAP)
Other recommended	• Doxorubicin, cisplatin, ifosfamide, and high-dose methotrexate

Guide 19
Second-line systemic therapy options: Osteosarcoma

Preferred options	• Ifosfamide (high dose) with or without etoposide • Regorafenib • Sorafenib
Other recommended	• Cabozantinib • Cyclophosphamide and topotecan • Docetaxel and gemcitabine • Gemcitabine • Sorafenib with everolimus
Used in some cases	• Cyclophosphamide and etoposide • Ifosfamide, carboplatin, and etoposide • High-dose methotrexate • High-dose methotrexate, etoposide, and ifosfamide Sm^{153}-EDTMP for relapsed or refractory disease beyond second-line therapy

Periosteal osteosarcoma

Periosteal osteosarcoma starts in the surface of the bone called the periosteum. Treatment is surgery to remove the tumor called wide excision. Chemotherapy might be given before surgery to reduce the size of tumor or the amount of cancer. Chemotherapy before surgery is sometimes called preoperative chemotherapy.

Low-grade osteosarcoma

Treatment for low-grade osteosarcoma is surgery to remove the tumor called wide excision. Chemotherapy might follow surgery if a high-grade component is found unexpectedly in the surgical specimen. Chemotherapy after surgery is sometimes called postoperative chemotherapy. Dedifferentiated parosteal osteosarcomas are not considered to be low-grade tumors.

High-grade osteosarcoma

This section is for high-grade osteosarcoma. Other types of high-grade non-osteosarcoma such as undifferentiated pleomorphic sarcoma (UPS) of bone could also be treated the same way.

Before surgery treatment

For most, treatment starts with preoperative chemotherapy. The goal is to shrink the size of the tumor before surgery. After chemotherapy, your cancer will be restaged to see if surgery is now possible.

Restaging

Imaging tests to restage your cancer might include:

- Chest CT
- MRI with or without CT (both with contrast) of primary site
- X-rays of primary site
- Consider PET/CT (head-to-toe) or bone scan

If tests find your tumor is unresectable, treatment will be radiation therapy or chemotherapy.

If tests find your tumor is resectable, treatment will be surgery to remove the tumor called wide excision. Treatment after surgery is based on if cancer was found in the surgical margin.

Treatment after surgery

Treatment after surgery is called adjuvant treatment. When no cancer is found in the surgical margin, it is called a negative margin. Treatment is chemotherapy. When cancer remains in the surgical margin, it is called a positive margin. Treatment might be chemotherapy, or more surgery. Radiation therapy might follow surgery, but it is rare. See Guide 20.

Metastatic disease

This section is for those with metastatic disease at diagnosis. Metastases can be found in the lungs (pulmonary), bone (skeletal), or internal organs (visceral). These are often resectable. Surgery to remove a metastasis is called a metastasectomy. Some metastases might be treated with systemic therapy, radiation therapy, or other therapies. For example, unresectable lung metastases might be treated with ablation.

If surgery is not possible, then the options are:

- Chemotherapy
- Radiation therapy

Guide 20
Treatment options after surgery: Osteosarcoma

Positive margins	Good response →	• Chemotherapy • Consider additional local therapy such as surgical resection with or without radiation therapy (RT)
	Poor response →	• Consider additional local therapy such as surgical resection with or without radiation therapy (RT) • Continue with same preoperative chemotherapy
Negative margins	Good response →	• Chemotherapy
	Poor response →	• Continue with same preoperative chemotherapy

Monitoring

After completing treatment, you will be monitored to watch for signs that cancer has returned called recurrence or relapse. Monitoring includes physical exam, blood and imaging tests, functional assessment, and regular visits with your orthopedist and oncologist. See Guide 21.

Relapse

If cancer returns, treatment is systemic therapy and/or surgery. Surgery is not always possible. Systemic therapy options can be found in Guide 19.

After treatment for relapse you will have the following imaging tests:

- X-ray
- CT and/or MRI (both with contrast)
- Chest CT with or without contrast

If your cancer has responded to treatment, then you will be monitored for the return of cancer (relapse) or for progression.

Treatment options for relapse and disease progression include:

- Surgery to remove tumor (resection), if possible
- Clinical trial
- Palliative radiation therapy (may include samarium)
- Best supportive care

Best supportive care is treatment to improve quality of life.

Guide 21 **Monitoring osteosarcoma**
Physical exam, imaging of primary site and chest (use same imaging as before)
Follow-up with orthopedist and oncologist: • Every 3 months for year 1 and 2 • Every 4 months for year 3 • Every 6 months for year 4 and 5, then once a year
CBC and other blood tests as needed
Consider PET/CT (head-to-toe) and/or bone scan
Reassess function every visit

Review

- Osteosarcoma is the most common type of bone cancer. It usually occurs in the thigh, upper arm, or shin.
- Treatment is a combination of therapies.
- After completing treatment, you will be monitored to watch for signs that cancer has returned called recurrence or relapse.
- Osteosarcoma can metastasize in the lungs (pulmonary), bone (skeletal), or internal organs (visceral). These are often resectable.
- A metastasectomy is surgery to remove a metastasis.
- Best supportive care is treatment to improve quality of life.

Did you know?

The terms "chemotherapy" and "systemic therapy" are often used interchangeably, but they are not the same. Chemotherapy, targeted therapy, and immunotherapy are all types of systemic therapy.

9 Making treatment decisions

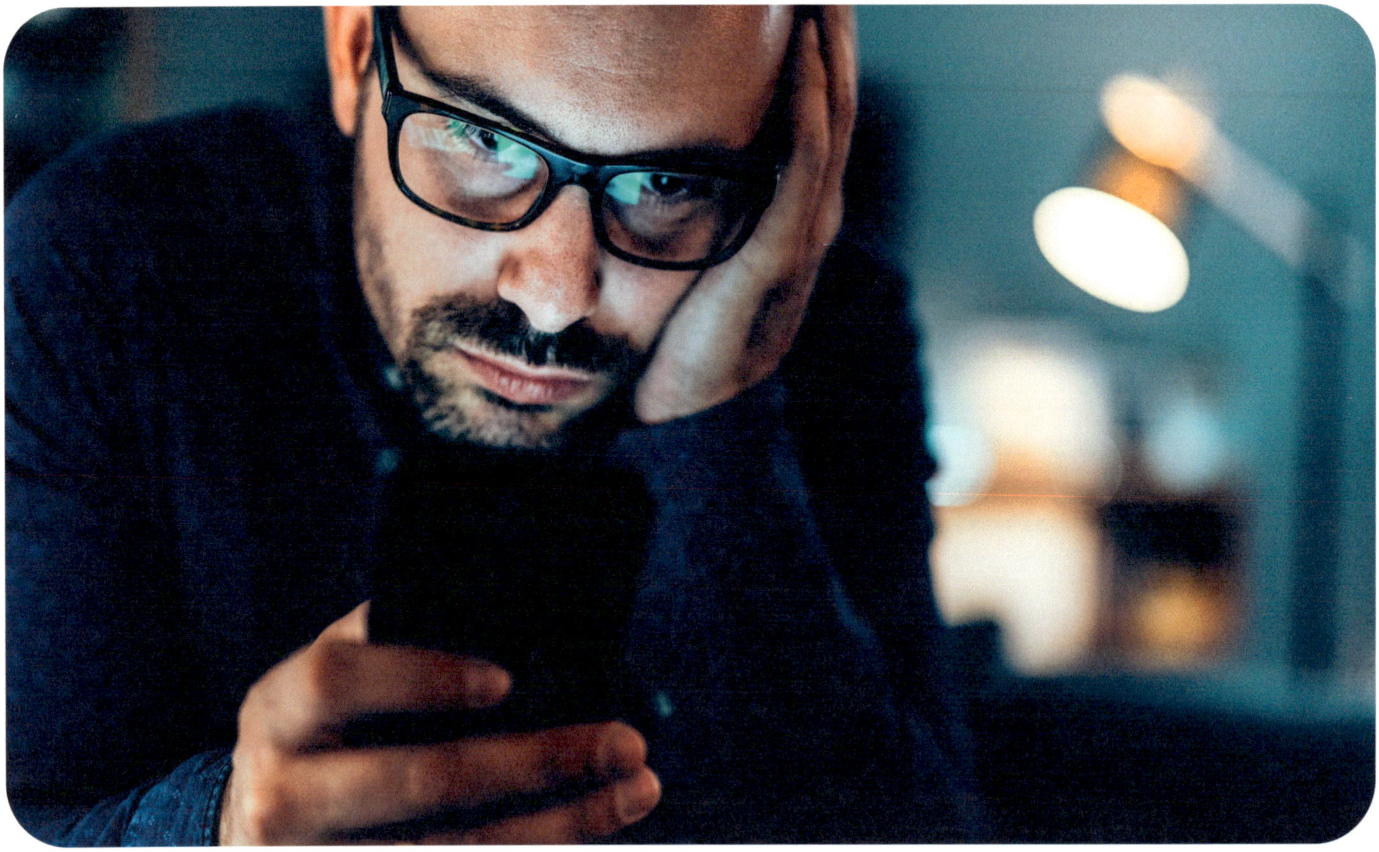

It's important to be comfortable with the cancer treatment you choose. This choice starts with having an open and honest conversation with your doctor.

It's your choice

In shared decision-making, you and your doctors share information, discuss the options, and agree on a treatment plan. It starts with an open and honest conversation between you and your doctor.

Treatment decisions are very personal. What is important to you may not be important to someone else.

Some things that may play a role in your decision-making:

- What you want and how that might differ from what others want
- Your religious and spiritual beliefs
- Your feelings about certain treatments like surgery or chemotherapy
- Your feelings about pain or side effects such as nausea and vomiting
- Cost of treatment, travel to treatment centers, and time away from school or work
- Quality of life and length of life
- How active you are and the activities that are important to you

Think about what you want from treatment. Discuss openly the risks and benefits of specific treatments and procedures. Weigh options and share concerns with your doctor. If you take the time to build a relationship with your doctor, it will help you feel supported when considering options and making treatment decisions.

Second opinion

It is normal to want to start treatment as soon as possible. While cancer can't be ignored, there is time to have another doctor review your test results and suggest a treatment plan. This is called getting a second opinion, and it's a normal part of cancer care. Even doctors get second opinions!

Things you can do to prepare:

- Check with your insurance company about its rules on second opinions. There may be out-of-pocket costs to see doctors who are not part of your insurance plan.
- Make plans to have copies of all your records sent to the doctor you will see for your second opinion.

Support groups

Many people diagnosed with cancer find support groups to be helpful. Support groups often include people at different stages of treatment. Some people may be newly diagnosed, while others may be finished with treatment. If your hospital or community doesn't have support groups for people with cancer, check out the websites listed in this book.

Questions to ask your doctors

Possible questions to ask your doctors are listed on the following pages. Feel free to use these questions or come up with your own. Be clear about your goals for treatment and find out what to expect from treatment.

Questions to ask about testing and staging

1. What type of bone cancer do I have? What is the cancer stage?
2. What is the grade of the cancer? What does this mean?
3. When will I have a biopsy? What type of biopsy? What are the risks?
4. Is there a cancer center or hospital nearby that specializes in this type of cancer?
5. What tests are needed? What other tests do you recommend? Will I have any genetic tests?
6. What will you do to make me comfortable during testing?
7. How do I prepare for testing? How and where will the test be done?
8. How soon will I know the results and who will explain them to me?
9. Is there a portal where I can get a copies of my test results and other records?
10. Who will talk with me about the next steps? When?
11. Will treatment start before the test results are in?
12. Can my cancer be cured? If not, how well can treatment stop the cancer from growing?

Questions to ask your doctors about their experience

1. What is your experience treating this type of bone cancer?
2. What is the experience of those on your team?
3. Do you only treat bone cancer? What else do you treat?
4. I would like to get a second opinion. Is there someone you recommend?
5. How many patients like me (of the same age, gender, race) have you treated?
6. Will you be consulting with experts to discuss my care? Who will you consult?
7. How many procedures like the one you're suggesting have you done?
8. Is this treatment a major part of your practice?
9. How many of your patients have had complications? What were the complications?
10. Who will manage my day-to-day care?

Questions to ask about options

1. What will happen if I do nothing?

2. How do my age, overall health, and other factors affect the options?

3. How will treatment affect my fertility? Should I see a fertility specialist before starting treatment?

4. What if I am pregnant? What if I'm planning to get pregnant in the near future?

5. Am I a candidate for a clinical trial?

6. Which option is proven to work best for my cancer subtype, age, and other risk factors?

7. Does any option offer a cure or long-term cancer control? Are the chances any better for one option than another? Less time-consuming? Less expensive?

8. Which treatment will give me the best quality of life? Which treatment will extend life? By how long?

9. What are our options if the treatment stops working?

10. Can I stop treatment at any time? What will happen if I stop treatment?

Questions to ask about treatment

1. Which treatment do you recommend and why? What are the benefits and risks?
2. How long do I have to decide?
3. Will I have to go to the hospital or elsewhere for treatment? How often? How long is each visit? Will I have to stay overnight in the hospital or make travel plans?
4. Do I have a choice of when to begin treatment? Can I choose the days and times of treatment?
5. How much will the treatment hurt? What will you do to make me comfortable?
6. How much will this treatment cost? What does my insurance cover? Are there any programs to help pay for treatment?
7. What kind of treatment will I do at home? What can I do to prepare my home to ensure my safety or the safety of other family members in the household? What type of home care will I need?
8. Are there any life-threatening side effects of this treatment? How will these be monitored?
9. What should I expect from this treatment? How long will treatment last?
10. How do you know if treatment is working? How will I know if treatment is working?
11. What in particular should be avoided or taken with caution while receiving treatment?

Questions to ask about surgery

1. What kind of surgery will I have? Will I have more than one surgery?
2. What will be removed during surgery?
3. Does my cancer involve any veins or arteries? How might this affect surgery?
4. What are the pros and cons of limb-sparing surgery versus amputation?
5. How long will it take me to recover from surgery?
6. How much pain will I be in? What will be done to manage my pain?
7. What other side effects can I expect from surgery? What complications can occur from this surgery?
8. What treatment will I have before, during, or after surgery?
9. Is there a hospital or treatment center you can recommend for my surgery?
10. How often will I need check-ups after surgery? What are the chances that the cancer will come back?
11. What happens if all of the cancer cannot be removed during surgery?

Questions to ask about radiation therapy

1. What type of radiation therapy will I have?
2. What will you target?
3. What is the goal of this radiation treatment?
4. How many treatment sessions will I require? Can you do a shorter course of radiation?
5. Do you offer this type of radiation here? If not, can you refer me to someone who does?
6. What side effects can I expect from radiation?

Questions to ask about clinical trials

1. What clinical trials are available? Am I eligible for any of them? Why or why not?
2. What are the treatments used in the clinical trial?
3. What does the treatment do?
4. Has the treatment been used before? Has it been used for other types of cancer?
5. What are the risks and benefits of this treatment?
6. What side effects should I expect? How will the side effects be controlled?
7. How long will I be on the clinical trial?
8. Will I be able to get other treatment if this doesn't work?
9. How will you know the treatment is working?
10. Will the clinical trial cost me anything? If so, how much?

Questions to ask about side effects

1. What are the side effects of treatment?
2. How long will these side effects last? Do any side effects lessen or worsen in severity over time?
3. What side effects should I watch for? What side effects are expected and which are life threatening?
4. When should I call the doctor? Can I text?
5. What medicines can I take to prevent or relieve side effects?
6. What can I do to help with pain and other side effects?
7. Will you stop treatment or change treatment if there are side effects? What do you look for?
8. What can I do to lessen or prevent side effects? What will you do?
9. What side effects are life-long and irreversible even after completing treatment?
10. What medicines may worsen side effects of treatment?

Questions to ask about survivorship and late effects

1. What happens after treatment?
2. What are the chances cancer will return or I will get another type of cancer?
3. Who do I see for follow-up care? How often? For how many years?
4. What should I do if I have trouble paying for follow-up visits and tests?
5. What tests will I have to monitor my health?
6. What late effects are caused by this treatment? How will these be screened?
7. I am looking for a survivor support group. What support groups or other resources can you recommend?
8. What happens if I move after treatment and have to change doctors? Will you help me find a doctor?

Websites

American Association for Clinical Chemistry
labtestsonline.org

American Cancer Society
cancer.org/cancer

Cancer*Care*
cancercare.org

Chemocare
chemocare.com

Children's National®
childrensnational.org

Children's Oncology Group
survivorshipguidelines.org

Chordoma Foundation
chordomafoundation.org

KidsHealth®
kidshealth.org

MedlinePlus
medlineplus.gov

Musculoskeletal Tumor Society (MSTS)
msts.org

National Cancer Institute
cancer.gov/types

National Coalition for Cancer Survivorship
canceradvocacy.org/toolbox/

National Hospice and Palliative Care Organization
nhpco.org/patients-and-caregivers

Northwest Sarcoma Foundation
nwsarcoma.org

OncoLink
oncolink.org

Radiological Society of North America
radiologyinfo.org

SARC
sarctrials.org

Stupid Cancer
stupidcancer.org

The Alan B. Slifka Foundation
slifkafoundation.org

The Paula Takacs Foundation
paulatakacsfoundation.org

The QuadW Foundation
quadW.org

Words to know

ablation
A procedure that uses extreme cold or extreme heat to destroy cancer cells.

biopsy
A procedure that removes fluid or tissue samples to be tested for a disease.

bone marrow
The soft, sponge-like tissue in the center of most bones where blood cells are made.

bone marrow aspirate
The removal of a small amount of liquid bone marrow to test for disease.

bone marrow biopsy
The removal of a small amount of solid bone and bone marrow to test for disease.

chemotherapy
Drugs that kill fast-growing cells, including cancer cells and normal cells.

chromosomes
Long strands that contain bundles of coded instructions in cells for making and controlling cells.

clinical trial
A study of how safe and helpful tests and treatments are for people.

computed tomography (CT)
A test that uses x-rays from many angles to make a picture of the insides of the body.

contrast
A chemical put into your body to make clearer pictures during imaging tests.

core needle biopsy
A procedure that removes tissue samples with a hollow needle. Also called core biopsy.

dual energy x-ray absorptiometry (DEXA)
A test that uses small amounts of radiation to make a picture of bones. Also called bone densitometry.

embolization
A procedure that treats tumors by cutting off their blood supply.

external beam radiation therapy (EBRT)
A cancer treatment with radiation received from a machine outside the body.

functional assessment
A test that looks at your ability to manage tasks and activities that are used in daily life.

hereditary
Passed down from parent to child through coded information in cells (genes).

hypercalcemia
Higher than normal levels of calcium in the blood.

gene
Coded instructions in cells for making new cells and controlling how cells behave.

grade
A rating of how much cancer cells look like normal cells.

immunotherapy
A treatment with drugs that help the body find and destroy cancer cells.

interventional radiologist
A doctor who is an expert in imaging tests and using image-guided tools to perform minimally invasive techniques to diagnose or treat disease.

magnetic resonance imaging (MRI)
A test that uses radio waves and powerful magnets to make pictures of the insides of the body.

medical oncologist
A doctor who is an expert in cancer drugs.

metastasis
The spread of cancer from the first tumor to a new site.

metastasectomy
Surgery to remove a metastasis.

monitoring
Testing after treatment ends to check for the return of cancer. Also called surveillance.

oncologist
A doctor who is an expert in the treatment of cancer.

ossification
Process of new bone formation.

osteoblasts
Bone-forming cells.

osteoclasts
bone-dissolving cells.

palliative care
Health care that includes symptom relief but not cancer treatment. Also sometimes called supportive care.

pathologist
A doctor who is an expert in testing cells and tissue to find disease.

positron emission tomography (PET)
A test that uses radioactive material to see the shape and function of body parts.

primary treatment
The main treatment used to rid the body of cancer.

primary tumor
The first mass of cancerous cells.

progression
The growth or spread of cancer after being tested or treated.

radiation therapy (RT)
A treatment that uses high-energy rays.

radiologist
A doctor who is an expert in imaging tests.

recurrence
The return of cancer after a cancer-free period.

refractory
A cancer that does not improve with treatment.

relapse
The return or worsening of cancer after a period of improvement.

remodeling
Process where bone cells are resorbed and new cells are formed.

resectable
A tumor that can be removed completely with surgery.

sarcoma
A cancer of bone or soft tissue cells.

soft tissue sarcoma
A cancer that starts in the cells of fat, muscles, nerves, tendons, blood and lymph vessels, and other supportive tissues of the body.

stereotactic radiosurgery (SRS)
A cancer treatment that uses special equipment to position the body and give one precise, large dose of radiation.

subtype
A smaller group within a type of cancer that is based on certain cell features.

supportive care
Health care that includes symptom relief but not cancer treatment. Also called palliative care or best supportive care.

surveillance
Testing after treatment ends to check for the return of cancer. Also called monitoring.

systemic therapy
Treatment that works throughout the body.

targeted therapy
A drug treatment that targets and attacks specific cancer cells.

translocation
When pieces of two chromosomes (long strands of coded instructions for controlling cells) break off and switch with each other.

unresectable
A tumor that cannot be removed with surgery.

NCCN Contributors

This patient guide is based on the NCCN Clinical Practice Guidelines in Oncology (NCCN Guidelines®) for Bone Cancer. It was adapted, reviewed, and published with help from the following people:

Dorothy A. Shead, MS
Director, Patient Information Operations

Laura J. Hanisch, PsyD
Medical Writer/Patient Information Specialist

Erin Vidic, MA
Medical Writer

Rachael Clarke
Senior Medical Copyeditor

Tanya Fischer, MEd, MSLIS
Medical Writer

Stephanie Rovito, MPH, CHES®
Medical Writer

Kim Williams
Creative Services Manager

Susan Kidney
Graphic Design Specialist

The NCCN Guidelines® for Bone Cancer 1.2021 were developed by the following NCCN Panel Members:

*J. Sybil Biermann, MD/Chair
University of Michigan Rogel Cancer Center

*Warren Chow, MD/Vice-Chair
City of Hope National Medical Center

Sarah Boles, MD
UC San Diego Moores Cancer Center

Brian Brigman, MD, PhD
Duke Cancer Institute

Alexandra K. Callan, MD
UT Southwestern Simmons Comprehensive Cancer Center

Lee D. Cranmer, MD, PhD
Fred Hutchinson Cancer Research Center/ Seattle Cancer Care Alliance

Saeed Dianat, MD
Abramson Cancer Center at the University of Pennsylvania

Eric Donnelly, MD
Robert H. Lurie Comprehensive Cancer Center of Northwestern University

Nicola Fabbri, MD
Memorial Sloan Kettering Cancer Center

Patrick Getty, MD
Case Comprehensive Cancer Center/ University Hospitals Seidman Cancer Center and Cleveland Clinic Taussig Cancer Institute

John Groundland, MD
Huntsman Cancer Institute at the University of Utah

Susan M. Hiniker, MD
Stanford Cancer Institute

Angela Hirbe, MD
Siteman Cancer Center at Barnes-Jewish Hospital and Washington University School of Medicine

Margo L. Hoover-Regan, MD
University of Wisconsin Carbone Cancer Center

Francis Hornicek, MD, PhD
UCLA Jonsson Comprehensive Cancer Center

Lisa Kafchinski, MD
O'Neal Comprehensive Cancer Center at UAB

Joseph B. Kuechle, MD, PhD
Roswell Park Comprehensive Cancer Center

Dieter Lindskog, MD
Yale Cancer Center/Smilow Cancer Hospital

David R. Lucas, MD
University of Michigan Rogel Cancer Center

*Joel L. Mayerson, MD
The Ohio State University Comprehensive Cancer Center - James Cancer Hospital and Solove Research Institute

Sean V. McGarry, MD
Fred & Pamela Buffett Cancer Center

*Carol D. Morris, MD, MS
The Sidney Kimmel Comprehensive Cancer Center at Johns Hopkins

Damon R. Reed, MD
Moffitt Cancer Center

Peter S. Rose, MD
Mayo Clinic Cancer Center

Victor M. Santana, MD
St. Jude Children's Research Hospital/ The University of Tennessee Health Science Center

Robert L. Satcher, MD, PhD
The University of Texas MD Anderson Cancer Center

Joseph Schwab, MD, MS
Massachusetts General Hospital Cancer Center

Herbert Schwartz, MD
Vanderbilt-Ingram Cancer Center

Breelyn A. Wilky, MD
University of Colorado Cancer Center

Rosanna L. Wustrack, MD
UCSF Helen Diller Family Comprehensive Cancer Center

NCCN Staff

Mary Anne Bergman
Guidelines Coordinator

Giby V. George, MD
Oncology Scientist/Medical Writer

* Reviewed this patient guide.

For disclosures, visit NCCN.org/about/disclosure.aspx.

NCCN Cancer Centers

Abramson Cancer Center
at the University of Pennsylvania
Philadelphia, Pennsylvania
800.789.7366 • pennmedicine.org/cancer

Fred & Pamela Buffett Cancer Center
Omaha, Nebraska
402.559.5600 • unmc.edu/cancercenter

Case Comprehensive Cancer Center/
University Hospitals Seidman Cancer
Center and Cleveland Clinic Taussig
Cancer Institute
Cleveland, Ohio
800.641.2422 • UH Seidman Cancer Center
uhhospitals.org/services/cancer-services
866.223.8100 • CC Taussig Cancer Institute
my.clevelandclinic.org/departments/cancer
216.844.8797 • Case CCC
case.edu/cancer

City of Hope National Medical Center
Los Angeles, California
800.826.4673 • cityofhope.org

Dana-Farber/Brigham and
Women's Cancer Center |
Massachusetts General Hospital
Cancer Center
Boston, Massachusetts
617.732.5500
youhaveus.org
617.726.5130
massgeneral.org/cancer-center

Duke Cancer Institute
Durham, North Carolina
888.275.3853 • dukecancerinstitute.org

Fox Chase Cancer Center
Philadelphia, Pennsylvania
888.369.2427 • foxchase.org

Huntsman Cancer Institute
at the University of Utah
Salt Lake City, Utah
800.824.2073
huntsmancancer.org

Fred Hutchinson Cancer
Research Center/Seattle
Cancer Care Alliance
Seattle, Washington
206.606.7222 • seattlecca.org
206.667.5000 • fredhutch.org

The Sidney Kimmel Comprehensive
Cancer Center at Johns Hopkins
Baltimore, Maryland
410.955.8964
www.hopkinskimmelcancercenter.org

Robert H. Lurie Comprehensive
Cancer Center of Northwestern
University
Chicago, Illinois
866.587.4322 • cancer.northwestern.edu

Mayo Clinic Cancer Center
Phoenix/Scottsdale, Arizona
Jacksonville, Florida
Rochester, Minnesota
480.301.8000 • Arizona
904.953.0853 • Florida
507.538.3270 • Minnesota
mayoclinic.org/cancercenter

Memorial Sloan Kettering
Cancer Center
New York, New York
800.525.2225 • mskcc.org

Moffitt Cancer Center
Tampa, Florida
888.663.3488 • moffitt.org

The Ohio State University
Comprehensive Cancer Center -
James Cancer Hospital and
Solove Research Institute
Columbus, Ohio
800.293.5066 • cancer.osu.edu

O'Neal Comprehensive
Cancer Center at UAB
Birmingham, Alabama
800.822.0933 • uab.edu/onealcancercenter

Roswell Park Comprehensive
Cancer Center
Buffalo, New York
877.275.7724 • roswellpark.org

Siteman Cancer Center at Barnes-
Jewish Hospital and Washington
University School of Medicine
St. Louis, Missouri
800.600.3606 • siteman.wustl.edu

St. Jude Children's Research Hospital/
The University of Tennessee
Health Science Center
Memphis, Tennessee
866.278.5833 • stjude.org
901.448.5500 • uthsc.edu

Stanford Cancer Institute
Stanford, California
877.668.7535 • cancer.stanford.edu

UC San Diego Moores Cancer Center
La Jolla, California
858.822.6100• cancer.ucsd.edu

UCLA Jonsson
Comprehensive Cancer Center
Los Angeles, California
310.825.5268 • cancer.ucla.edu

UCSF Helen Diller Family
Comprehensive Cancer Center
San Francisco, California
800.689.8273 • cancer.ucsf.edu

University of Colorado Cancer Center
Aurora, Colorado
720.848.0300 • coloradocancercenter.org

University of Michigan
Rogel Cancer Center
Ann Arbor, Michigan
800.865.1125 • rogelcancercenter.org

The University of Texas
MD Anderson Cancer Center
Houston, Texas
844.269.5922 • mdanderson.org

University of Wisconsin
Carbone Cancer Center
Madison, Wisconsin
608.265.1700 • uwhealth.org/cancer

UT Southwestern Simmons
Comprehensive Cancer Center
Dallas, Texas
214.648.3111 • utsouthwestern.edu/simmons

Vanderbilt-Ingram Cancer Center
Nashville, Tennessee
877.936.8422 • vicc.org

Yale Cancer Center/
Smilow Cancer Hospital
New Haven, Connecticut
855.4.SMILOW • yalecancercenter.org

Index

Made in the USA
Monee, IL
05 November 2026

67385763R00052